The Golden Boy

HAWORTH Gay & Lesbian Studies
John P. De Cecco, PhD
Editor in Chief

New, Recent, and Forthcoming Titles:

Gay Relationships edited by John De Cecco

Perverts by Official Order: The Campaign Against Homosexuals by the United States Navy by Lawrence R. Murphy

Bad Boys and Tough Tattoos: A Social History of the Tattoo with Gangs, Sailors, and Street-Corner Punks by Samuel M. Steward

Growing Up Gay in the South: Race, Gender, and Journeys of the Spirit by James T. Sears

Homosexuality and Sexuality: Dialogues of the Sexual Revolution, Volume I by Lawrence D. Mass

Homosexuality as Behavior and Identity: Dialogues of the Sexual Revolution, Volume II by Lawrence D. Mass

Understanding the Male Hustler by Samuel M. Steward

Sexuality and Eroticism Among Males in Moslem Societies edited by Arno Schmitt and Jehoeda Sofer

Men Who Beat the Men Who Love Them: Battered Gay Men and Domestic Violence by David Island and Patrick Letellier

The Golden Boy by James Melson

The Golden Boy

James Melson

Harrington Park Press
An Imprint of The Haworth Press, Inc.
New York • London • Norwood (Australia)

ISBN 1-56023-015-0

Published by

Harrington Park Press, an imprint of The Haworth Press, 10 Alice Street, Binghamton, NY 13904-1580

Library of Congress Cataloging-in-Publication Data

In respect for their privacy, the names of many individuals appearing in *The Golden Boy* have been changed.

Melson, James, 1957-1992
    The golden boy / James Melson.
      p.   cm.
    ISBN 1-56023-015-0 (acid-free)
    1. Melson, James, 1957-1992 – Health. 2. AIDS (Disease) – Patients – United States – Autobiography. I. Title.
RC607.A26M456 1992
362.1'969792'0092 – dc20
[B]   91-36061
                                                                     CIP

CONTENTS

Foreword   vii
     Lawrence D. Mass

Preface   xvii

Chapter 1: Childhood in Sundown Town   1

Chapter 2: A Star Is Born   11

Chapter 3: Higher Education   23

Chapter 4: Iowa Boy in the Windy City   35

Chapter 5: "New York Is Where I'd Rather Stay"   51

Chapter 6: Moving Up in the World: Cape Cod   89

Chapter 7: Rubbing Elbows with the Rich and Famous   105

Chapter 8: The Model Student   117

Chapter 9: My Son, the Banker   139

Chapter 10: The Not-So-Innocents Abroad   161

Chapter 11: Nikos   175

Chapter 12: The Big A   189

Epilogue   211
     Arnie Kantrowitz

Foreword

Many homosexuals are obligatory narcissists.

— Lawrence Mass

In 1980, James Melson was The Golden Boy. Young, blond, beautiful, and gay, he was a regular at Studio 54, Flamingo, and other citadels of New York's high life in the heyday of the sexual revolution. Vain, hedonistic and politically unconscious, he was, in the vernacular of the day, a narcissist.

In January of that same year, I published my first piece for *Christopher Street*, a cover-story critique of *The Culture of Narcissism*, Christopher Lasch's patriarchal indictment of the younger generation. Entitled "The New Narcissism and Homosexuality: The Psychiatric Connection," my essay explored the popularity of the voguish nomenclature of *narcissism*, its basis in a new psychiatric category of mental illness called the "narcissistic personality disorder," and the psychiatric conceptualization of homosexuality as a phenomenon of "pathological narcissism." Here was my argument:

> *Are* homosexuals narcissistic? Is there indeed some truth to what . . . an entire psychiatric and psychoanalytic tradition has been saying about homosexuality for more than fifty years? Yes — the same kind of truth that labels blacks as sociopathic and of inferior intelligence because of their higher crime, unemployment and illiteracy rates. Many homosexuals are obligatory narcissists. Deprived of role models, of social structuring, of identity, constantly ridiculed, threatened, punished and endangered for natural sexual instincts, homosexuals have been completely excluded (not unlike women) from honest participation in the partriarchal societies they have lived in . . . . The "narcissistic" self-absorption that so many homo-

sexuals exhibit may actually be among the most extraordinary examples of human adaptability in the face of adversity . . .

This, I believe, is the larger context in which to appreciate James Melson's story. Like so many of us, the author was raised in an America that was profoundly ignorant and mendacious about all aspects of sexuality, especially homosexuality. Melson's upbringing in Dubuque, Iowa, wasn't so unlike my own, in Macon, Georgia and later, Chicago, where Melson lived briefly during his college years. For us, homosexuality was the deep, dark secret that could not be discussed, betrayed or even secretly owned. We had no idea who we were.

I was born in 1946. In 1959, I was carrying on with Richard H., a friend from school. We'd stay over at each other's homes on weekends, a widely tolerated adolescent/teenage practice that parents still don't recognize as a major opportunity for sexual exploration because they don't acknowledge the sexuality of their children. After sex one night, Richard turned to me and asked: "Do you think we're homos?"

"No," I said. At 13, I knew virtually nothing about "homosexuality"—a term that carried such stigma it couldn't even be printed in mainstream newspapers until the mid-1960s. The only time I'd ever seen the word was in one of my father's medical textbooks, published in the mid-1950s and oozing the most virulent "psychopathic personality" homophobia of the day. As a child, I had crossdressed and was always attracted to boys, but I was also attracted to girls. Richard and I both dated, excelled in sports and were well regarded among our peers, so I knew we weren't "homos"—the "queers" and "sissies" who were alternatively ostracized, jeered, or otherwise victimized at school—or like the people in the medical freaks book. But I had no idea what our desires and experience did mean and there seemed to be no way of finding out. My one "sissy" friend (one of those designated as such by most of our classmates), who later became a rich closet case, was in much greater denial about his sexuality than Richard, who later married and raised a family. Meanwhile, I knew of no older, respected person who was like me, who I might talk to, and it would be another year before I would begin reading novels like *Auntie Mame*,

Giovanni's Room, and *Our Lady of the Flowers* in pursuit of understanding.

Although born 11 years later, Melson had a parallel experience. At 13, he first considered the possibility that there were others like him when he noticed that Blake, one of the regulars at the Dubuque Golf and Country Club, was

> rail thin and flawlessly coiffed and sprayed by Duane's Villa de Coiffure . . . [and] would lounge with [the ladies] at pool's edge for hours on end, deciphering whose husband was sleeping with whose wife and who was seeing a shrink . . . . Despite our ridiculing poor, obvious Blake and his glamorous poolside pose as swinging single and ladies' man, I was fascinated by him, his devotion to self-beautification and his mysterious private life. Who were his male friends? . . . Blake would appear on the tennis courts with a short muscleman, also single, but very masculine. Surely *he* couldn't be queer . . . or could he? . . . It would be years before I had rid myself of stereotypes about homosexuals, and about all sorts of other minorities as well.

It was 1975. Melson was 18 and was about to be introduced to his first gay bar, though he did not yet know that "gay" was subculturalese for homosexual. Meanwhile, with no role models, no social context in which to identify himself, no counseling, no lover, he proceeded with "my first true love: the mirror."

I didn't enter my first gay bar until I was 20. By 1975 (I was 29), however, my progress was such that I had come out to my family. In the throes of my first real love affair—with a man twice my age—I had come out to my father in 1969. He wished me well. My confession didn't unhinge his faith in my abilities as a physician, though he warned that I would eventually be "found out." Patriarchally skeptical of my mother's ability to deal with such adult fare, he advised me not to tell her. But Mom figured it out, and she did so with perfect timing, just after the American Psychiatric Association declassified homosexuality as a mental disorder in 1973-74.

If Melson had been ten years older in 1975, would he have been more socially conscious and connected to the gay movement that was emerging around him? Is it unreasonable to wonder why, even at the tender age of 18, he had no awareness of the APA declassification? Unfortunately, it would take a diagnosis of AIDS before this personification of so much of the gay culture of his time would become political, and even then, the transformation was largely unwitting. It commenced when his illness forced him to come out to his family and progressed with his decision to come out to the world in the writing and publishing of his autobiography.

Larry Kramer concludes his book, *Reports From The Holocaust: The Making of an AIDS Activist*, with his account of a confrontation between his sister-in-law and himself. This breaking down of the barriers of communication between your significant others and yourself, Kramer seems to be saying, is where politicization begins—i.e., the personal is political. It is this transformation that makes Melson's story of historical interest. That it takes place so reluctantly and tacitly also makes it literary and gives it a dimension of tragedy.

In 1980, Melson was moving in exclusively gay circles, but none of his fuck-buddies, lovers, roommates, and co-workers had any political consciousness. They were denizens of the world of Larry Kramer's novel, *Faggots*, published in 1978. Like AIDS, the gay movement is in the background of Melson's experience. There is no mention of any demonstrations, of Larry Kramer, his novel, or his later pieces on AIDS: no mention of gay pride parades, the assassination of Harvey Milk, the Masters and Johnson or Kinsey studies of homosexuality, Rock Hudson, Liberace, Leonard Matlovich, Harvey Fierstein, AIDS and gay movement cover stories in leading publications, or of homophobia in the media. Instead, Melson details the star-spangled night life he fell into at Studio 54 and other watering holes of the "beautiful people."

Not that I couldn't identify with Melson. I went to some of the same pleasure palaces, did some of the same drugs, and was "promiscuous" (a word I always placed in quotes because of its enormous abuse in the mouths and by the pens of critics of the gay liberation movement and the sexual revolution). My youth and looks (I was the swarthier, chunkier type) gave me entrée to grand estates and exclusive resorts. But I became more aware of my minority identity, more disenchanted with the selfishness, self-destructiveness, cruelty, and homophobia of the so-called beautiful people, especially those who were gay (I had known Larry Kramer since the late 1960s and knew and/or had slept with some of the characters so mercilessly flayed in *Faggots*). As I entered my thirties and the invitations to beachfront homes in the Hamptons and Pines began to dwindle, I got more involved. In 1979 I did my first pieces for the gay press — a history of my experiences coming out during interviews for a residency in psychiatry (*Gay Community News*), an interview with Masters and Johnson, and a review of their book, *Homosexuality in Perspective (The Advocate)*, as well as an overview of the academic literature on sadomasochism *(The Advocate)*. The year 1980 saw the first issue of the *New York Native*, in which I had a feature on homophobia in film. In 1979 and 1980, the first medical reports were published of cases of Kaposi's sarcoma in gay men, which would later be understood to be AIDS-related. In 1981 I became the first writer to cover the AIDS epidemic in any press (mostly in the *Native*).

There was a big difference between Larry Kramer's and my own reactions to the James Melsons of 1970s gay culture. In the years surrounding the publication of *Faggots*, I would still see Larry, my senior by more than a decade, at the baths, but Larry was never a very happy or successful fast-laner, as his novel attests; despite considerable success as a screenwriter, he wasn't regarded as one of the "hot men" by the fast-lane types he pursued and hadn't succeeded in finding a lover. Is that why he had never participated in gay movement organizations or demonstrations, many in the community wondered? When his brilliant satirical novel, *Faggots*, was universally condemned by the politically correct types as homophobic, erotophobic, and treasonous, he became even more bitter and resentful, and nearly all of his anger was directed at the gay community rather than at the homophobic society-at-large, which gay liberation spokespersons of the day held one hundred percent responsible for all gay troubles. Still involved in fast-lane gay culture as well as the fledgling gay liberation movement when *Faggots* was published, and, not so unlike Melson, grateful for all the fun and love I'd had, I felt a lot more affirmative about my life, to the point (very unlike Melson) that I became extremely concerned about and protective of "my people" and "my children" (as I thought of

them and as Larry would later refer to us in speeches). Even now, I
have compassion for the politically unconscious types. I don't hate
them. It's a real challenge, but I don't even hate the many rich and
professionally successful gay "friends" I've had, the closet cases
who still don't have an iota of consciousness, who have never lifted
a finger to help out, either in the movement or during the epidemic;
the "friends" whose only politics were their pocketbooks, who financed right-wingers, who wouldn't contribute a penny to any gay
cause, and who, adding insult to injury, often had contempt for
those of us who were fighting for *their* civil rights! As I still see it,
their self-hatred is mostly a by-product of gigantic forces of homophobia and oppression. Like self-hating Jews, closet cases be-
tray their victimization. Even when they have nothing to lose — like
Roy Cohn and Terry Dolan on their deathbeds — they cannot be
honest or generous. They are deeply disturbed. Of course, *some* of
these people are truly evil and cause enormous damage. I'm an
ardent admirer of Michelangelo Signorile and am deeply sympathetic with the outing movement, just as I believe Jews who collab-
orated with the Nazis should have been and should be publicly identified, vilified, and prosecuted; but *most* closet cases, like most
self-hating Jews, merely lack insight and courage and are more pathetic than hateful or genuinely tragic. In attempting to come to
terms with his experience, however superficially and unsuccess-
fully, Melson becomes tragic in a way that Dolan and Cohn, who
were profoundly hateful and who never showed any insight or re-
morse, did not. Beneath Melson's star-struck account lies the irony
that so many of the famous people he names or alludes to, especially the fashion moguls, met our earliest appeals for funds for the
disease he died of with slammed phones and doors.

Larry Kramer was absolutely fed up with a community whose
hedonism he saw as the cause, rather than a consequence, of all its
troubles, and when we came together to form Gay Men's Health
Crisis in 1981-82 (around the time Melson developed a case of shingles), there were numerous clashes about leadership and the tone of
our appeals to the community. As a physician, I believed that the
epidemic needed to be covered as accurately as possible. As a gay
activist, I believed that the messages needed to be conveyed as sex-
affirmatively as possible, that we needed to be exceedingly careful

not to throw the baby of gay civil liberties out with the bathwater of an STD epidemic that, in perspective from the beginning, had nothing more to do with gay people *per se* than syphilis had to do with Jews (who were episodically scapegoated for its spread in Europe). As a proud and self-identified member of the gay community, I believed our message would be most successfully targeted if it came from community and/or movement leaders and heros. Most of the earliest members of GMHC were, in fact, James Melson types — beautiful boys who had never been involved in the gay movement, who led closety lives at work, and spent their summers in Fire Island Pines. But it was there that many of those who were being kept by rich aunties had gotten to know a man they revered as, hands down, the most virile of their kind, the daddy of their fantasies; a man who was also the most respected and beloved among them. That man was Paul Popham, co-founder and first president of Gay Men's Health Crisis. This incredibly handsome, former Green Beret, whose speaking voice had the raspy sexiness of Michael Bolton's singing, had a charismatic effect on gay men, despite his shyness. Because his decency and generosity were an easy match for his looks, that effect was also salutary. There can be no question that to an enormous extent, GMHC's earliest success in achieving credibility, attracting support, and reaching its target population was the direct result of Paul's leadership and hard work.

Unfortunately, Paul was also politically conservative. He had no experience with public affairs and had never been any kind of activist. The extent to which he gave himself to the community that had worshiped him was truly heroic, and his achievement was nothing less than the basic structure and functioning of what was to become the largest and most prominent organization in the history of the gay liberation movement; but more radical approaches were needed. Instead of working *with* Paul, however, Larry Kramer brutally and incessantly attacked the organization and its leadership for all that it wasn't doing. In this case, I believe that Larry, who is otherwise so unquestionably the premiere and supreme hero of the AIDS epidemic, was wrong, notwithstanding the power of his attacks to motivate his enemies, who more often than not were community leaders. (Larry's perspective is detailed in his play, *The Normal Heart*. My perspective is further elaborated in *Homosexuality and Sexual-*

ity: Dialogues of the Sexual Revolution, Volume I, The Haworth Press, Inc., 1990.) What was needed all along was a second organization to do the political work that GMHC was never set up to do. When Larry finally realized this in the mid-1980s and founded ACT-UP, his attacks on GMHC did not cease, but they diminished in direct proportion to ACT-UP's success. Instead of expending so much primary time and energy going after GMHC and the gay community, he finally turned full-force to the true villains — the government, the FDA, the Republicans, closet cases with power who were actively thwarting our progress, etc.

Whatever our differences, Larry and I were in agreement on the most important points, like the seriousness of the epidemic and the extent of ignorance about sexually transmitted diseases in our community and the world at large. Melson's story documents this reality. In the late 1970s, Melson, in his twenties, saw his first uncircumcised penis and didn't know what it was (he thought the glans was missing). Although Melson finally mentions KS and AIDS by name, there's no awareness of the STD epidemics in the gay community that immediately preceded AIDS: hepatitis B, syphilis, gonorrhea, and amebiasis. With such people in mind, Larry wanted the information about the epidemic to be conveyed in the simplest do-and-don't terms. In *The Normal Heart*, Ned Weeks (the Kramer character) asks Dr. Emma Brookner what to tell the community. "Tell gay men to stop having sex," she says. That's what Larry wanted us to blare as widely and loudly as possible. On the other hand, I argued, there were a lot of intelligent and concerned members of the community who wanted to know specifics. Should the new proscriptions include "wet kissing"? Handholding? "Stop having sex" seemed just as vague and unacceptable a solution then as it does today — as unrealistic an approach to the epidemic as "Just Say No" (the title of Kramer's satirical play about the Reagan era) is to the drug crisis. Of course, both approaches — the simplistic and the nuanced — were necessary, but neither was to reach Melson. His only connection with a gay organization comes at the end of his story, when he mentions attending an AIDS support group.

The debate about AIDS education and its failure, in any form, to touch the lives of countless James Melsons, highlights another important perspective Larry and I fought over from the earliest days of the epidemic: the medical historical experience that great epidemics are not solved by behavioral approaches, even if such approaches may save individual lives, but by successful treatments (e.g., as with antibiotics for syphilis and gonorrhea) and vaccines (e.g., polio). In my interview with then acting New York City Health Commissioner David Sencer (*New York Native*, 1/31/83), this perspective was articulated:

> *Mass:* At the Mount Sinai symposium on AIDS last July, you said that behavioral approaches to the control of AIDS were likely to be relatively ineffective. As was the case with polio, the real solution will be a preventive vaccine or its equivalent. Am I accurately describing your thinking about AIDS?
>
> *Sencer:* Let's go back to polio. We recognized early on that the method of spread was oral-fecal. An individual could do certain things to minimize her or his risk. They could stay at home, they could avoid communal swimming, crowded places, etc. Individuals may have minimized their risk in some cases with such measures. But the real control of polio came with the development of a preventive vaccine.

Eight years later, in his keynote address at the Gay Men's Health Crisis Memorial Service, "A Gathering of Remembrance and Renewal" (at the Cathedral of St. John the Divine, 11/22/91; as reprinted in *The Village Voice*, 12/10/91), Larry Kramer drew the same conclusion:

> I don't believe anymore that education works, and we're putting so much trust in it. Education did not stop Magic Johnson from getting AIDS. Nor Kimberly Bergalis . . . . The figures are marching inexorably faster than we can ever stop them by education . . . . The only thing that is going to make this plague go away is a cure at the most and successful treatments at the least . . .

Because AIDS is caused by a virus, and there are no known cures for viruses, Larry's prediction needs to be modified in only one regard: While we must continue to look for cures and successful treatments, the most realistic hope for bringing an end to this epidemic is a preventive vaccine, as with smallpox and polio. Meanwhile, how vividly *The Golden Boy* demonstrates this truth about the limits of preventive education.

As we await a vaccine and/or cure, where, then, do we stand today, in 1992, a decade into what may already be the greatest epidemic in recorded history? In the last chapter, Melson chronicles the losses, ostracisms, and indignities that begin to snowball with the advance of his disease. At the airport, he is approached by a black heroin addict, Jenny Moses, begging for money. He gives her five dollars and then shares a snack with her. They promise to pray for each other. "I hopped back on the Carey bus with a smile on my face," he says, "happy about helping the poor waif with something to eat and a few hopefully inspiring words." In this encounter, which is as close as Melson comes to self-transcendence, is the whole universe of the personal as political. Indeed, in the communion of these unlikely bedfellows lies the future of the epidemic and the world politics in which it is so increasingly and inextricably entwined.

– Lawrence D. Mass
New York City, 1992

Preface

When I was diagnosed with AIDS in 1985, I cut a deal with God. I asked him to allow me to do the following before he takes me: (1) further develop my relationship with Him, (2) sail in Nantucket, (3) travel the rocky coast of Maine in the peak of autumn foliage, (4) come to grips with and make amends for the selfish, self-centered person I've been all my life, (5) go to Southern California (where I now live), and (6) most importantly, finish my book. Well, it's my fifth year with full-blown AIDS, and as you'll see, I've accomplished all that I set out to do. As I half-jokingly tell my friends, I now am ready to reserve a seat (first class of course) on the Trump Shuttle to heaven. Despite everything I was before, I think the past five years have left me worthier of my wings. But of course, that won't be for me to decide.

I am dedicating this book in honor of—and I thank God for—these few people who have remained staunch friends, and whom I love so dearly: Tim, Cindy, Keith, Norm, P-nut—and especially Marti, for without her help the completion of this book would not have been possible. I am also dedicating it to all those who are presently coping with the scourge of AIDS, as well as those who have lost the fight.

Jim Melson
1991

Chapter 1

Childhood in Sundown Town

I was born in America. I will live an American. I shall die an American.

—Daniel Webster

Dubuque, Iowa, also known as Sundown Town, is a redneck, rough-shootin' meat packing town on the Mississippi River at the juncture of Illinois, Iowa and Wisconsin. The population is roughly 60,000, of whom 80 percent are Catholic. (However, Dubuque was long devoid of racial diversity: It was well known that if a black man hit town looking for a job, he would be approached by police "suggesting" he be gone by sundown.)

On September 7, 1957, Greta Elizabeth Melson, age forty, gave birth to James Kenneth, myself; a beautiful, tow-headed, ten-pound baby boy—the product, I maintain, of a frisky New Year's Eve romp. My parents claimed I was "planned," and not a "mistake." BULLSHIT! In any event, given my mother's age it's safe to say I made it just before menopause.

My mother was born in Alborg, Denmark. In 1922, at age five, she emigrated to the U.S. with her mother Torah, sister Irsa and brother Finn. Torah decided to emigrate after my grandfather, a concert violinist, had an affair with a young protégé. There was a divorce, and after news of the whole business got around, my grandmother could no longer hold her head up in public.

At the time, an immigrant to the U.S. had to have a relative who was a U.S. resident sign on his or her behalf, as a sponsor. Torah's brother Eklund, who worked for the Danish government in Saint Croix, Virgin Islands—a territory of the U.S.—was to meet her as

1

she got off the boat at New York's Ellis Island. He was nowhere to be found. A wire arrived saying he had been taken ill with tuberculosis and could not make the trip from St. Croix. My grandmother was mortified — what would she do stuck in New York with three children? She had sworn she would never return to Denmark as long as she lived. One of her few U.S. acquaintances, an old flame named Henry with whom she had corresponded over the years, worked in Detroit for the Ford Motor Company. She called him and explained her predicament. Still single, and still madly in love with Torah after some ten years, he immediately traveled to New York. They were married, immigration was granted, and my grandmother settled down with Henry Erik Jensen in Detroit. Predicament solved!

When the Depression hit, Henry was laid off from his job indefinitely. Spending her teens deprived of material comforts we take for granted today, my mother acquired a shrewdness with money which she retains even today, despite the extremely comfortable bounty supplied by my father. (After all, one never knew when disaster might once again hit and all would be lost.) For instance, during a recent visit home I opened a kitchen cabinet and was buried by an avalanche of soda cans which she saves for redemption at five cents apiece. She scolds me for calling information for phone numbers instead of using the book.

My father Kenneth (Kenny) was born in Osage, Iowa, also to Danish immigrants. His father owned and operated the local grocery store until he lost it in the Depression. An alcoholic, my grandfather died from cirrhosis of the liver prior to my birth. My grandmother Christine, who recently died at age ninety-eight, had always been a crotchety old thing, which explains my father's general coldness, toughness and lack of sensitivity. She wouldn't give the time of day to her grandchildren, either. As a child, when we would visit, I would hide out in the nooks and crannies of her Osage attic apartment, coming out only for her homemade apple pie: that was absolute heaven. But I thought she was a bona fide reincarnation of the Wicked Witch of the West, reminiscent in looks, voice and demeanor of Margaret Hamilton in *The Wizard of Oz*. Children were to be seen and not heard. "Spare the rod and spoil the child" was her credo. "A good whacking is healthy from time to time . . .

makes men out of boys." Torah, on the other hand, used to bounce me on her lap, singing Danish children's songs. Aside from lack of parental love, Kenny grew up fighting tooth and claw with his five athletic brothers for the number one spot in everything. The end result of this upbringing was a hard-driving, hard-drinking, charismatic success; the consummate man's man.

Dad's life consisted of dawn-till-dusk meat hawking. Dusk brought major martinis — extra dry, extra olive — with the boys at one of Dubuque's innumerable bars and taps. My father loved to identify himself as one of "them" — the workers. Although totally devoid of pretense in the conventional sense, he would, with each drink, soar into a loathsome, braggadocious monologue about his self-made success, and then was usually driven home by a less inebriated companion to unload his finale on my mother and me. He combined the self-confidence of Kirk Douglas with the humor of a lower-brow Johnny Carson. His taste in food was strictly meat and potatoes: Sauces, he considered emasculating; casseroles, women's bridge club fare. Eating out was either at Bucky's Steak and Rib Joint, or not at all.

My mother's life, on the other hand, was filled with bridge clubs, charity work and crafts. She was one of the "ladies who lunch," or as close as you could get in Dubuque. Evenings were usually spent separately, with father ensconced in his den in front of the TV, watching war movies, football, cop dramas, anything violent. This was undoubtedly the result of his jocky upbringing. No one would cross a Melson. Mother remained in the kitchen either knitting or doing crossword puzzles while watching Englebert Humperdink and Tom Jones on TV.

My brother Eric was my idol as a child. Fifteen years my senior, he could be both generously loving and horribly mean to me. For my birthday he once built me a train set, with mountains, houses and factories. He made snowslides at the side of our house for me and my little aluminum flying saucer; and one Christmas morning I got a beagle puppy tied with red ribbon, which Eric had coaxed my mother into buying and which I named Toto. Thanks to him, Santa had finally brought me a puppy of my very own. His cruelty, on the other hand, manifested itself in various ways: blowing up my sandbox with a cherry bomb while I was in it; grabbing my fat belly with one hand and lifting me up mid-air (he called this the "Texas claw"); approaching me with hands clenching, releasing, clenching, releasing, sending me running screaming bloody murder to my mother.

One year when he was playing baseball with friends, I begged him to allow me to join in. They were all age sixteen and up. I was five or six. They finally relented and said, "Okay, Jimmy, you can play," and told me to lie down on the dirt. Not knowing anything about the game, I lay down and eagerly awaited their next instruction. The pitch was made, the ball was hit and the batter ran to first base and came sliding into me at second. I was the second base.

Regardless, I loved him; he was my father figure, as my father was too busy with his work and drinking with pals to deal with another child. I remember him telling my mother once, "Greta, you raise the kid till he's thirteen and then I'll take over and give him the balls and guts to handle life." Little did he know that for a child, emotionally, it doesn't work that way. Children do not switch on love and respect like a circuit breaker after being ignored for thirteen years.

I was six years old when I discovered my fascination for Ken dolls. Soon after, the G.I. Joe dolls came out. The smooth, muscular plastic body made my little legs tremble, made me crazy with desire. I begged my parents for one for my seventh birthday. Although at that age I had no idea what sexuality even was, I definitely appreciated a fine human form.

My father's back went out on him during that period and my mother bought him a hand vibrator. Thanks to my neighbor playmate, I soon discovered a different use for the item. When either of our parents were out, we would call each other, get together and satiate our prepubescent sexual hungers. A game we used to play with a third friend was "gorilla." One of us would play the gorilla, the other two, zoo visitors. The gorilla would escape from his cage and the visitors would pretend to faint. The gorilla would then bring out the vibrator and have his way with us. Then we would regain consciousness, not remembering a thing; a good time, with an easy way out of our guilt. Thanks to moms and dads, all three of us knew that playing with peepees was bad. Still, that was no deterrent. The forbidden activities continued until the day white stuff came out. I thought I had contracted some deadly disease as God's punishment for my sexual misbehavior. My parents had seen no need to tell me the facts of life. Pregnancy was not an issue for boys. Let the girls worry about it: if they missed their periods, they were whores. The boys responsible were studs. Girls would usually disappear from school into Hillcrest Home for Unwed Mothers. Due to the 80 percent Catholic composition of Dubuque, abortion was unheard of as an alternative.

Despite my raging (if bizarre) sexual activities, my childhood grew increasingly painful. My earliest painful memory is from my first grade class's weekly show-and-tell. When my week came, I really wanted to impress everyone. I'd spent the preceding days combing my mother's dresser for Danish mementos to use as props for telling the story of my Danish heritage. Thursday morning I carried in a shoebox full of miniature Danish flags, a violin pick of my grandfather's, an old pipe, and a tiny statuette of Hans Christian Anderson's Little Mermaid.

As "curtain time" approached, my stomach started to rumble. I could feel it coming. I raised my hand for permission to go to the bathroom, but couldn't get Mrs. Martin's attention. What was I going to do? I couldn't hold it. Finally . . . blasto, diarrhea for days. I sat stonefaced, searching for some way out of the mess but there was no escape. Mrs. Martin turned from the board to call me up to the front for my presentation. I shook my head no. "Come up here, Jimmy, and bring what you have." I told her I forgot. Unfortunately, the box was on the floor next to my desk, clearly in view. "Your box is on the floor, now get up here immediately."

"I can't."

With that Mrs. Martin marched down the row of seats to my desk, grabbed hold of my ear and pulled me out of my desk and up to the front as diarrhea slid down my legs and onto the floor. The class looked on. There was a moment of total silence; then hysterical laughter followed by a united chorus of "Jimmy pooped his pants, Jimmy pooped his pants." I was sent to the nurse's office to change into a nurse's gown and wait for my mother to pick me up. I was humiliated beyond any hope of recovery.

I always had a love for sweets. Beginning at age eight, I ballooned into quite a mass of flesh. At thirteen, I was five feet tall and weighed one hundred eighty-five pounds. My mother was unfortunately a pre-Dr. Spock type: "Eat everything on your plate, Jimmy, or no dessert." I would, of course — and then stuff myself with one or two butterscotch sundaes. Then on to my father's Oreo cookies, etc., etc., etc. Needless to say, the extra poundage did not help foster my social life. From age ten on, dealing with girls was impossible. I tried flirting, but was constantly shunned due to my appearance. With boys it was worse. Sports were of paramount importance in my hometown. I was extremely uncoordinated, so instead of practice, I would usually walk the long road to home (and TV) alone — until I met Bobby. He was even fatter than I and much shorter. His cheeks were so enormous they looked as if they would explode at any minute, and his thick-lensed horn-rimmed glasses made his squinty eyes look like eight balls. Soon Bobby was walking (or waddling) me home; we became soulmates, and above all, foodmates.

Two places would tempt us en route: First, the Milk House — a country-type store with a large glass-enclosed bakery display case full of glazed donuts. I would fight with Bobby over first choice, always dictated by the amount of tooth-rotting sugary glaze. Armed with donuts, Bobby and I would continue on our food odyssey. Next stop was White's grocery store for cakes and cookies. After all, boy does not live on donuts alone. Soon home, we would check out the refrigerator and beg our mothers for something to eat; well, we were starved from the long walk home! This daily pig-out was really disgusting. I usually stole my donut money from Mom's purse the night before. At the time, school lunches were forty cents each. Extra items were available at extra charge. My mother would give me forty cents every morning, but I usually had much more from my previous night's thievery. Lunch was my favorite meal of the day, especially if they had the highly coveted, spectacularly delicious apple crisp. I made sure I had lots of extra change on those days.

Nevertheless, I was extremely depressed most of the time, as I sank further and further into fat. My 36 to 38 inch-waist pants were constantly splitting. My extracurricular activities and hobbies were limited to the constant search for confectionary bliss.

Gym class on Tuesdays and Thursdays became a horror story.

Two ex-Marine-type coaches with hair shaved close to their heads played favoritism with the athletes while I was the constant target of humiliations that would scar me for life. One time we were being tested for our skills on the trampoline. There were two trampolines in the gym, one brand new, the other simply prehistoric, with frayed, worn elastic bands and an unresponsive spring. Most of the kids would go on the new trampoline; I, on the old. All the kids would come over to watch my fat jiggle while I bounced. The poop man was now Jello Jimmy. When it was my turn to be tested, I prepared to do some dramatic move such as a seat drop: I gave it my all in the jump, and my feet and legs went right through the criss-crossing elastic bands of the tramp. It was as if I had trapped myself in a giant diaper—as though to add the coup de grâce to my previous disgrace. My chaffed and scraped legs dangled, unable to touch the floor. The coaches told a couple of the kids to get up on the tramp to weigh it down and stretch the elastic bands, so someone could get underneath and push my legs back up through the holes. Instead the kids started jumping and laughing, while I sat stuck in my "diaper" bouncing helplessly as a paddleball. Finally, the coaches called in the janitors to cut the bands. When they did, I thudded to the floor like a tub of lard. More hysterical laughter and name calling from the other kids.

Compounding the stigma of my weight was the fact that I was the last in my class to go through puberty. In the locker room, while the other kids proudly exposed their growing members and sprouting bushes in vainglorious style, my minuscule acorn-like peepee was a source of pain and insecurity. My fat, pink rear end became the target of every towel-snapper. "It's the eunuch! The fat poopy eunuch!" I just couldn't take it. Showers were mandatory; I would try my best to sneak out showerless, but the coaches would usually catch me and send me back, snapping towels at me themselves. (*Et tu, Brute!*)

For two long years this was my nightmare. Finally, at thirteen, my day of reckoning came. My parents went to the Orient for a month-long vacation, and enlisted a couple of college students to watch the house and cook for me. "Cooking for me" turned out in short order (so to speak) to mean fixing a peanut butter or bologna sandwich on Wonder bread—or at any rate, something so unappetizing that I would usually pass it on to my little dog Toto. They would go out someplace for dinner and spend the grocery money my parents had provided on themselves. I had forty cents a day for my lunch, but without my mother's purse, how was I to supply my apple crisp and donut supplements?

I remember studying myself naked in my mother's full-length dressing room mirror one night, and bursting into tears. Between what there was to see — my sallow, white skin, the disgusting rolls of fat — and what there was to *eat*, the truth was clear and inescapable: it was diet time.

During the remainder of my parents' absence I literally starved myself. I simply went to the other extreme. I ate only celery and carrot sticks. I was determined to become thin and hopefully well-liked and admired. I lost twenty-five pounds in those few weeks. At the same time, puberty finally kicked in, and my metabolism shifted from first gear into overdrive. The fat melted off. The less I fed my stomach, the more I fed my yearning for a beautiful, athletic body like those of the jocks at school who had tortured me daily. My rear end would no longer be used for target practice. I would show them.

I went along to the airport to pick up my parents on their return. My mother got off the plane and walked right by me, not recognizing me at all. When I called out to her and she finally realized it was me, tears welled up in both our eyes simultaneously. She was so proud of me, and for the first time in my life I was proud of myself. No longer was I the fat boy of the class and never would I be again. I was consumed with the willpower I never knew I had.

Aside from my gorilla episodes, my earliest experience with a true-to-life homosexual was at my parents' country club, which was my stomping ground in my youth. Between the pool and baby pool were lounge chairs and umbrellas where middle-aged women would tan, gossip, count each other's cellulite pockets, and sip their refreshments — usually something pink and innocent-looking, but loaded with booze. As the afternoon went on, they would slowly get plowed in preparation for their husband's complaints about a dirty house, the evening's dinner and the lack of clean underwear. One of the regulars was Dolores Dixon, a pudgy widow with overly frosted hair, pale pink lipstick and dark glasses — the then-fashionable Liz Taylor look. Dolores usually parked herself on one of the chaises with Blake Gallagher. Blake was an heir to Dubuque's Gallagher Furniture Company fortune. His primary purpose in life seemed to be to challenge George Hamilton for the gold medal in the suntan Olympics. Rail thin and flawlessly coiffed and sprayed by Duane's Villa de Coiffure, Blake would lounge with Dolores at pool's edge for hours on end, deciphering whose husband was sleeping with whose wife and who was seeing a shrink. His suntan oil was spread so thick, the glare could penetrate the darkest of Ray-Bans. One day, as my fellow junior high schooler and aspiring gossip Peggy Hauser and I watched this couple only yards away in peak chatter, Peggy suggested I use the pool phone to have Blake paged. Although I knew Peggy to be a troublemaker from birth, the temptation was irresistible. With minimal coaxing from her Pippy Longstockingish grin, I proceeded to the phone and dialed the club number. I heard a pompous "Dubuque Golf and Country Club." "I'd like to page Blake Gallagher at the pool, please."

"Certainly, sir, please hold."

I hung up and scurried back to our perch to wait. Within seconds, "Blake Gallagher, line five-eight, line five-eight" sounded over the loudspeaker.

Blake jerked upright, gasping, "God, Dolores, it's him!" and swivelled daintily to the phone. He pushed button after button, getting nothing but the dial tone. Peggy and I were fit to explode with laughter as Blake poured out obscenities. On the verge of tears, he retreated to Dolores for consolation.

Despite our ridiculing poor, obvious Blake and his glamorous poolside pose as swinging single and ladies' man, I was fascinated by him, his devotion to self-beautification and his mysterious private life. Who were his male friends? Who did he expect to find at the other end of the phone line, and what did he and whoever it was do together? Blake would appear on the tennis courts with a short muscleman, also single, but very masculine. Surely *he* couldn't be queer . . . or could he?

It would be years before I had rid myself of stereotypes about homosexuals, and about all sorts of other minorities as well.

Chapter 2

A Star Is Born

Some men see things as they are and say "why?" I dream of
things that never were and say "why not?"

—Robert F. Kennedy

I entered Dubuque Senior High School in September, 1971, and
began what was to be a wonderful, formative experience for both
my body and mind. One would not expect miracles from a public
high school in Redneck City, but it was a real birth to me. I continued to be shunned by the jocks, despite my weight loss, but was
quickly accepted into the theater group. The fall play was Molière's
A Gap in Generations; I auditioned for the role of Dr. Graziano, a
character of high comedy and gross eccentricity who looms large in
the cast. In preparation for the audition I had perfected a cackling,
henlike voice and teased my fairly long blond hair up into a frizzy
mop. When Fran, the drama coach, announced the parts and named
me for Dr. Graziano, my spirits soared. At long last I felt the prestige and status which came naturally to other students (or which
they enjoyed by virtue of *their* extracurricular activities). The
drama group was highly admired in the school. Except possibly for
the cheerleaders, its girls were the prettiest of all; its boys a bit fey,
but hysterically funny.

However, my self-image had not yet adjusted to my weight loss.
Psychologically I was still the fat boy. I was terrified of opening
night: Would it be the old story—everyone laughing at Jello Jimmy's feeble attempts at accomplishment—that is, at *me* rather than
at Dr. Graziano? Or, on the other hand, would there merely be
stony silence just when everyone should be rolling on the floor?

Always having been a loner, and unused to interaction with others, I would now be judged by perhaps hundreds. How would I get through this—me, an insignificant nothing? What if I fouled up? This was my big chance, and here I was—a wreck. This self-torment went on throughout the rehearsal period.

On the big night, just before curtain time, Fran came up to me. She was an extremely perceptive woman, fully aware of the scars of my past humiliations, and of my present fears. She put her arms around me and told me what a fantastic job I'd done throughout the rehearsals and reassured me not to worry, Dr. Graziano would come through with flying colors. The curtain went up and as I spoke my first line, laughter roared from the audience. All my fears dissolved, and being on stage felt totally natural. I couldn't even see the audience in the darkness beyond the footlights; only their laughter came through; and the more they laughed, the more it brought out the ham in me—the *lean* ham that had clearly been inside the fat pig, trying to get out. When the curtain came down and the cast came out on stage for bows, I was the last; the applause roared with three curtain calls and a standing ovation. I was on top of the world, wishing the applause would go on forever.

I was to rest on my theater laurels for quite some time to come. The performance gave me immediate and widespread recognition among teachers and students alike. A new body, and stardom, all in one year; it was too much. I was convinced I was Hollywood bound.

After my brief triumph, I became obnoxiously cocky within the theater group. I did Readers Theater and state speech contests, and was admitted into the Thespian Honor Society; but no more major roles. Fran became fed up with the prima donna I had become. My self-assumed star quality had gone to my head, and alienated not only her, but the rest of the group as well.

My new-found self-confidence and transformed looks, and the fact that my father was Senior Vice President of Dubuque Packing Company (also known as 'the Pack'), the largest privately owned meat packing company in the country, gained me entrée into the "in" group. My fat-boy image had vanished. My new friends were doctors', lawyers' and bankers' kids; privileged, intelligent and good-looking, not to mention snobby and snotty. We were an amazingly pretentious and materialistic group, all deserving of a major ass-whacking, and spent most of our time bar-hopping, playing poker, smoking pot, lighting farts and talking about chicks. (*Just* talking.) My best friend, however, continued to be Mort Smith, whom I had met long before in my Cub Scout troop. Mort was funny-looking, with big lips, squinty eyes and buck teeth. The more brutally prejudiced kids insinuated, with their charming wit, that Mort was the progeny of "a Geisha whore raped by a nigger." The mutual pain we had experienced bonded us together for life; misery loves company. Mort's parents were talented, good-looking and socially prominent. In fact, he felt so overshadowed by his parents' success that he avoided any serious attempts at achievement for fear of failure. Like me, he was uncoordinated in sports and so had no interest. He had a good wit, but it wasn't enough to overcome his loser complex. Mort was the only person that I was better than at almost everything, which wasn't saying much, but which still gave me great pleasure. I lorded it over him. He always fought back, but that only added to my enjoyment. Our quarrels always blew over; for the most part we were inseparable.

Mort's neighbor was Ed Russell, also in our class. Ed was dark and good-looking with hairy legs, the sight of which gave me goose bumps and made my penis harden. Having grown up as country club babies, all three of us decided to go out for the school swim team. Practice was from seven to nine in the morning and after school from four to six. It was grueling, but it was the third major factor in my physical metamorphosis (the first being my crash diet during my parents' trip, the second, the onset of puberty). I had lost 45 pounds in just a matter of months. The transformation was so dramatic and so ego-gratifying that I couldn't walk past a mirror, or store window — indeed, anything reflective — without checking myself out. Before dinner I would disappear into my mother's dressing room to gaze, enraptured, at the same mirror that only a short time before had displayed a disgusting mass of fat, but that now offered the image of a handsome young man. It was a classic "mirror mirror on the wall" fairy tale come true. This was my first true love: the mirror.

Whereas before, my future had seemed nothing more than a long slide into a tub of lard, now anything seemed attainable. My destiny seemed almost divine. I was *special*. For my tortured youth, I had at long last been justly rewarded with a face and body. Now what to do with them? Although I was a poor swimmer, the mere fact that I joined the team added to my prestige and social standing at school. Mort, however, couldn't hack it and soon dropped out. Ed was a superb diver. After our laps, I would watch him practice, displaying amazing precision, toes pointed and heavily muscled legs flexing wildly as he hit the boards. Ed had a beautiful body, with a washboard stomach and a promising basket in his tight Speedo suit — all of which he flaunted. He was number one in the class academically and state diving champion to top it off. By virtue of all this, but this alone, he had become one of "the group." Girls swooned over Ed; they all wanted him for his achievements and his good looks; as they watched him on the boards, young pussy would moisten and gush. But he was socially inept, boring, and seemingly oblivious to their attention.

Skiing further strengthened my friendship with Ed. Once he invited me to accompany him and his family to ski for the day at Chestnut Mountain Resort, across the Mississippi near Galena, Illinois. (Here, "mountain" is something of a euphemism: Comparing the hills of the Midwest to, say, the mountains of Colorado is like comparing Olive Oyl to Dolly Parton.) Skiing was my favorite sport. While I enjoyed swimming, I dreaded the races, especially losing — which I usually did — then getting out of the pool, shivering, next to naked, and walking to the locker room with my tail between my legs. Skiing was a different story. Eventually I started to race in the NASTAR and collected numerous medals; another boon to my ego.

Knowing how much I loved the sport, my father had a discussion with Ed's father — an extremely talented architect, but, like Ed, a social dud — about developing a ski area on the Iowa side of the Mississippi. But there was big money involved. After a lot of thought, and with much reluctance and my persistent begging and pestering, my father (who didn't even ski) wrote Mr. Russell a check for $10,000 dollars as an initial investment.

I was elated. We would actually own part of a ski resort. The redneck kids would turn green-necked with envy, and I would lord it over them in sweet retribution. The resort would be called Sundown. Seven families were involved. For financial reasons, initially the families did all the work themselves. The group was composed of businessmen and professionals who had the necessary expertise — an engineer, an architect, the owner of a well and pump company, and so on — except for my father; all he had was a few extra bucks. Still, he was a trooper and all-around contributor — fumbling with the construction of a garage door for the lodge, for example, while cussing extravagantly in true Melson style. A thorough lack of mechanical ability was one of the very few things he and I had in common. (The operative question would surely have been, "How many Melsons does it take to screw in a light bulb?")

Kenny's sports interests lay in hunting, fishing, and contact sports. Skiing wasn't manly enough. If there weren't blood and guts spilled or heads bashed, he considered it a woman's sport. Skiing had become a rich man's sissy sport, not much more masculine than ballet. Why, when *he* was a kid, he and his brothers strapped barrel staves to their shoes and headed out to Osage's old Cedar River bluffs. (Exaggerated tales of childhood deprivation were my father's stock in trade.) None of these newfangled, down-filled get-ups in designer colors for old Kenny! Winters would later bring my father out to the hill, but in a ragged hunting coat — like some Hemingway of the slopes — and then only to look over his investment. Obviously, his motive for the investment wasn't his enthusiasm for the sport, nor was it purely financial; rather, it seemed to be his way of making up for my earlier "life without father."

Work was slow, drudgerous and physically exhausting. A few of the slope areas were open fields, but most were covered with thick, prickly cedar trees. These had to be felled with chain saws and dragged down to the bottom of the slope. It seemed we would never get through. The chain saws were good for about an hour until sap got into the machinery and jammed up the cogs. The real excitement was dynamiting the hills. Tremendous amounts of limestone were blasted out and had to be carted away or deposited at slope bottom. At mealtimes the families and other workers gathered at the top of the hill under a large open tent. The food was always delicious; the mothers took turns preparing it and each tried to outdo the others. One day they made chocolate cream pies for dessert. The manager who had been hired for the resort, a huge bear of a man, had one too many beers and started a tremendous food fight with the cream pies and everything else. A torrential rainstorm soon followed, and the whole affair turned into a gigantic mud bath. We were all rolling in laughter and mud and food. As there were no showers for miles, we hosed each other off with ice-cold water. The incident became part of the Sundown group's lore, and contributed to the growing bonds between the various families — as only a good food fight will.

The Russells were a hardy group, and often we would make a fire and camp overnight at the hill in order to start work at dawn the next morning. Ed and I were out alone one night. It was so tranquil: the music, the fire, the lights of romantic Dubuque in the distance. We drank a few beers and discussed our aspirations and thoughts about life. Ed wished to attend medical school eventually. (I had no idea yet what I wanted. Academically I was a jack of all trades — competent in most subjects but master of none.) Night brought out the cool air. We got into our sleeping bags — his an expensive Eddie Bauer goose-down number that could have made a night in Antarctica uncomfortably warm; mine an old cotton and wool army bag. I began to freeze during the night and poked Ed to ask if he wouldn't mind sharing his bag with me. He agreed and I got in with him. Ed was quickly snoring. His pants were off and his hairy, muscular legs radiated heat. I was fascinated by those legs; I longed to reach down and rub my hands up and down their muscular silkiness. I soon mustered the guts to move my leg over to his, actually touching his hairy calf. I was getting very excited. He continued to snore. I became erect and I slowly moved it towards his leg. Ed Russell, state diving champion: what a hot jock this was! My sexuality was rising at last — and with a vengeance. I couldn't stop at touching his leg with mine; I found his penis with my hand. He, too, was hard, although he continued to snore. I stroked it long and slow. I couldn't believe it: I actually had a hard penis in my hand. It was wonderful. I was afraid he would wake up at any minute and beat the shit out of me; but he came almost immediately without awakening. (Or at least so I thought.)

Sundown opened the following February. The first week was only for the families, friends, workers and press. It was the culmination of all our work. A job well done. We were all very proud.

Now all it had to do was make money! The first year was a little rough, and the partners were squeezed to put more money in. They barely broke even that year, but each year thereafter the hill proved to be a money factory. It is now one of the largest and most successful resorts in the Midwest, especially popular among Chicagoans.

During the summers I took my annual job as a lifeguard at the country club, whose amenities I took full advantage of. There were lots of breaks during the other guards' shifts when I could play tennis or cards, swim, or just lie in the sun. I developed a beautiful golden tan, and my hair turned a whitish blond. And what with working out at a health club in town, swimming, and running on a country road near my parents' house, my body, which a mere two years before had been a disgusting mass of fat, was now hard and lean. The "handlebars" of my childhood had totally disappeared. I had blossomed into quite a beauty . . . or beauty queen. Girls in bikinis passed by my chair constantly, struttin' their stuff and aiming their charms my way. For the most part — and to their chagrin — I pretty much ignored them, good, conscientious lifeguard that I was.

More like, flaming narcissist that I was. At home, I would enter my mother's dressing room, still oiled from the pool, and masturbate to my own reflection. For post-masturbatory pleasure, I would go into my mother's makeup drawers and use her mascara and eyebrow pencil to create George Hamilton-like beauty marks and Cary Grant-like chin clefts — so totally enamored was I of my transformation. But how on earth had this happened? Would it last? Was I dreaming? Would I wake up and find myself a 195-pound butterball again? During the spring semester we had studied ancient history; nude, muscular marble sculptures abounded on every page — Adonis, Narcissus, Hercules . . . was I perhaps a reincarnation of one of them? While my body had developed, it was obvious that my psyche had developed too — into quite a sick piece.

During the spring term of my senior year, the French and German Clubs organized a trip to Canada. (The original goal was Europe, but the take from bake sales and car washes had fallen somewhat short.) Many of my friends went along, a good portion of whom had never been beyond the tristate area, not to mention the U.S. "Frère Jacques" rang through the bus — and rang, and rang, getting so tiring (truly "dormez-vous") by the time we hit Rockford, Illinois that "99 Bottles of Beer on the Wall" came as almost welcome relief. Mort and I sat together, with Ed behind. Ed had sent me a letter earlier in the spring informing me how revolted he was with the Sundown camping episode, and that we should remain friends, but not in bed. I was mortified. How could I possibly have believed he'd slept on while I was whacking off his meat?

A bathroom stop and seat change landed me next to Tammy Phillips. Tammy was a cheerleader from an "other-side-of-the-tracks" type of family. She had an angelic, roundish face, full lips, a heart-melting smile, beautiful white teeth, long brown hair, nice big tits and a perfect, tight ass. Needless to say, she was rather popular with the boys, and got constant come-ons and propositions from the jocks. For this, the other girls awarded her such endearing but undeserved titles as slut, tramp, whore, and anything else that envy of her sex appeal could inspire. Envy, hell: hatred.

We talked, joked and laughed most of the afternoon. As we crossed the Canadian border, the sun dropped and it got chilly. At Tammy's suggestion, we covered ourselves in a blanket. It was nearly dark, and under the blanket, we were hidden from anyone's view. I found myself reaching for her hand. She squeezed it gently — my cue to carry on. I undid her button-down blouse and slid my hand along her smooth stomach and slowly up to her breasts. As I began to massage her tits I could feel them swell. Her nipples felt the size of tollhouse cookies. So this is what a girl felt like! It was great! Nothing could have pulled my hands off her boobs. Meanwhile she masterfully unzipped my pants and slid her hand over my wet, engorged penis. She looked at me, smiled, and coyly feigned going to sleep — but didn't stop the strokes. It was a déjà vu of my experience with Ed. I was quick to come. Her lips curled upward in a sly smile but her eyes remained closed. I was a bit nervous about this undercover activity on the bus, but in the pitch dark, no one noticed a thing.

After about fifteen minutes our horniness was rearoused. Tammy took my hand and guided it down to her now unbuttoned jeans. I thought of Ed Russell. Suddenly, it was his protruding member I wanted, not some wet, juicy hole. Suddenly I felt terrified. I pulled my hand away and whispered to Tammy that I was tired. But perceptive as she was, I believe she knew at that moment that I was queer. No one had ever turned down Tammy's pussy. Never having tried anything with a woman prior to this, the episode also confirmed to *myself* that I was a homosexual. Only this time, the realization seemed genuine and it gave me pause. What would I do with my life? People hated homosexuals. Would I every marry? Hardly, unless "she" was gay as well. Would I turn out like Blake Gallagher? Suddenly, I felt lonely. I wanted a man, at least to have sex with. Although with Tammy I felt a tinge of romance, a gleam of something special, this was just not "it" for me.

Senior year zoomed by. It was a year full of achievement and recognition, but also of anticipation of and trepidation about my first semester of college. Would I be smart enough? Could I hack it? Who would my friends be? As the spring semester progressed it was time to start thinking about *which* college. Consultations with guidance counselors were scheduled and I was assigned a spinster in her late sixties about whom rumors abounded that she'd molested male students during their sessions with her. As I entered the reception room outside her office, I shuddered at the thought of wrinkled hands groping me and withered lips pressing against mine.

The door creaked open. "James, come in, please," she said. The sweetness of her voice and smile instantly banished my fears. She sat me down and said that, though I'd indicated I was interested in a large university in a major city, I should reconsider: Large universities tend to regard their students as numbers; I might not get the personal attention I was used to, coming from Dubuque Senior High School. "Your parents can certainly afford to send you to a quality private institution, James. I have one in mind: With your Scandinavian background, St. Olaf would be perfect for you. It's in a beautiful, tranquil community, Northfield, Minnesota, an hour's drive from Minneapolis and St. Paul; the campus is atop Manitou Heights and is beautiful; and the student body comes mostly from good Scandinavian families like yours. You're a good student James, but your grades don't quite qualify you as Ivy material. I suggest you think seriously about St. Olaf."

My guidance counselor must once have been a hypnotist or hawked swampland in Florida, because I was sold instantly. "Atop Manitou Heights" . . . it sounded so supreme . . . looking down on humanity. It seemed like poetic justice after my last ten years of misery. I would be surrounded by rich beautiful blonds. In ten years' time, I would be a demigod, holding court at my high school reunion, bragging about my success to classmates who had gone to Iowa State ("Moo U") or the University of Iowa, or ended up married and saddled with screaming children and nagging wives and working overtime at "the Pack." This would be my revenge for their years of abuse.

In early September my parents drove me up from Dubuque and helped me unpack my humble belongings while others were unloading stereo systems of forklift proportions. Goodbyes were said, tears were shed, and their little boy was cut from his umbilical cord.

Right from the outset, St. Olaf was everything my guidance counselor had promised. Architecturally it was a wonder: ivy-covered limestone walls, copper and slate roofs, giant oak doors and leaded mullioned windows set into elaborately carved granite frames; some of the buildings were copies of Norwegian castles. I truly felt closer to heaven on that hill—first, simply because of its elevation above the town, and second, from the sight of handsome, muscular Scandinavians unloading belongings from their parents' Mercedes, Volvos and Saabs. (For Dubuquers, Cadillacs, Lincoln Continentals or Chrysler Imperials were the epitome of the luxury automobile. These strange-looking foreign jobbies had never been flashy enough to elicit my admiration—not until Laura Beth Pendleton, ex-homecoming queen, debutante and glamourpuss in training from the posh Minneapolis suburb of Edina, casually mentioned the shocking five-figure amount that Daddy had forked over to a dealer for his 280 Sportster.)

I had never seen so many blond beauties gathered in any place at once in my life (and I'd seen some beauties to reckon with). Far from the blue-blazered prep-school types I'd expected, most wore hiking boots, turtlenecks, and Icelandic sweaters (which were "in" that year—the earthier the better); a relief, in view of the snobbishness and pretentiousness I had braced myself for. While I fell short in the stereo-system department, in personal appearance, at least, I would easily fit in.

For my major I chose economics, reasoning that that might be the most useful and marketable degree when it came to pursuing the career in business that my parents had always encouraged. (Even a casual mention of an interest in the arts, I feared, would have suggested I was a homosexual.) But with my poor track record in math, I should have known another route would have been more suitable. I didn't stop to think that calculus, trigonometry and statistics would be required. It was a struggle from day one. I got through with mostly B's, and barely passed calculus with a D, despite all my shmoozing with the professor. I was consistently at the back of his class, not only figuratively but literally: I always sat well to the back to escape the vile smell of his armpits, as he whipped off equations about as decipherable as Egyptian hieroglyphics. Whether I would ever get my degree at this rate was a question worthy of the sphinx.

Chapter 3

Higher Education

A bachelor never quite gets over the idea that he is a thing of beauty and a boy forever.

— Eleanor Rowland

Initially, my social life centered around the traditional hazing antics of a college freshman: mooning the girls' dormitories, setting the water tower on fire, streaking, etc. Not that we shirked our studies: there was much to learn — about shots of tequila with beer chasers; pot; coke. This last was never mentioned, for fear our fathers would find out we were doing the white stuff and cut us off from the green stuff. I, too, feared disownership, although in my case the fear was mostly that he would discover my sexual predilection.

After flunking out of the University of Iowa the first semester, Mort moved to Minneapolis to work at a small radio station, in a menial position no doubt created as a favor owed to his father by some business associates. On weekends I would take the bus up there to visit him. We'd go to the movies and the University of Minnesota bars, get drunk on beer and stoned on pot. One night Mort and I were downtown on Hennepin Avenue with another friend. I was dying to go to the bathroom. Mort pointed out a bar across the street called the Gay Nineties. Well, incredibly enough — or perhaps not — *this* kid from Dubuque still did not know, in that year of 1975, what that name meant, and what waited behind the door. Mort and his friend waited out in front. I went in and found myself amidst a large crowd. There were lots of handsome men who soon encircled me like hungry sharks. Not many women, I thought. One, however, was standing next to me — an exotic black woman in an evening gown and high heels. Just as she flashed me a smile of pearly whites, a young, fey boy with a Dorothy Hamill hairdo approached her from behind and whipped off her wig. S/he let out a loud, high-pitched, campy scream and took off after the merry prankster. Poor, mortified me! *A drag queen!* As I waded through the crowd toward the dance floor, the revelations continued to unfold. It was full of men dancing with men, some cheek to cheek and others kissing. I was flabbergasted—yet fascinated. I knew, but I guess I didn't really *know*, that there were others like me, Mort and Blake Gallagher. I wanted to stay, but I knew Mort and his friend would be waiting outside to enjoy a hearty laugh at my shock. My instinctive (or rather, conditioned) response was to protect my pride by playing it straight—and outraged. I went out, grabbed Mort by his shirt collar, called him a fag and told him how disgusted I was with the scene. It worked; the boys seemed genuinely embarrassed and apologetic. In retrospect, however, I would have done just what they had done had the situation been reversed and I'd had the guts to reveal myself as Mort just had.

I went back to Mort's apartment to spend the night before returning to St. Olaf the next day. We talked at great length that night. I asked him how he managed without sex throughout high school. "The Julien Hotel," he explained. The Julien Hotel was a sleazy, decaying structure on lower Main Street in Dubuque. There was a dark smoky bar to the right of the lobby. Basically, it was a hangout for a bunch of closeted, dirty old men. Mort would go into one of the bathroom stalls and wait. Soon another man would enter the next stall. There was a hole in the wall between the stalls. It was "show and tell" time. Mort would take the man's penis through the hole and frantically beat it off. Positions were then reversed and the other man would reciprocate. The men themselves never saw each other or spoke. This was the tragically clandestine existence of a homosexual in Dubuque. If found out, they would be victimized throughout Sundown Town: shamed by their families, damned by their church and ridiculed by their friends and by society at large. This would have been my fate too if I hadn't suppressed my desires for so long. Alas, much the same went for St. Olaf. The repression that reigned there kept those Nordic-god-like students at a tantalizing, agonizing distance, fueling my suppressed desires further. Everyone knew who dated whom, what parties one went to, who screwed whom, etc. My social life began to stagnate. I felt like a caged animal. Once ridiculed as a fat child, now I was intimidated by my peers because I could claim no sexual conquests. The Gay Nineties haunted me. I had to go back.

One Friday night I boarded the bus to the Twin Cities, my thoughts fixed on that bar. Mort was to meet me for a movie and dinner. It was an enjoyable evening as we drank ourselves into a stupor and reminisced of good times in high school. We cabbed up Hennepin Avenue back to Mort's, past the Gay Nineties and the prostitute district. Sleep was impossible as I wondered what my first real gay social experience would be like the next night. The next day I told Mort I had to return to school to prepare for an exam on Monday. At six o'clock in the evening I left. It was early for the night life, so I took in a movie, checked into a bargain-rate Days Inn motel, then went back out and walked around downtown, drifting toward the Gay Nineties. It was dark now. I stationed myself at a bus stop across the street, watching the line begin to form outside the bar. I walked slowly toward it in mounting fear and guilt. Good God, what if my parents ever found out? My friends at school? Would I be slandered? Blackmailed? Beaten up?

The bar got very crowded; moving through it was push and shove. Most of the crowd was seedy-looking — undesirables, I would have called them. The smells of smoke, sickening cologne and sweat hung oppressively. I quickly found a dark corner to hide and observe. I was uptight about talking to anyone until I saw a man standing alone at the bar, holding a drink. Relaxed and totally at ease, he contrasted with the twirling queens on the dance floor. Very Italian-looking, with a thick mustache and hairy arms, he was my physical opposite (I was hairless — my childhood crypto-sexual fantasy was the wolfman); and I was instantly attracted. He began moving towards me, and my heart leapt. He stood next to me for a while, without looking at me, then turned, smiled, and said, "What's going on?" I began to tell him about my life as a student, which should have bored him to tears, but he seemed genuinely interested. His name was Tony. He was an airline steward (then much more than today a highly coveted occupation, along with hairdresser, florist, and makeup artist, among young homosexuals

who lost themselves too readily in the gay subculture at the expense
of their academic and career ambitions). Nevertheless, he intrigued
me. An airline steward: Think of all the ports of call, the diverse
and constantly changing array of men!

The conversation continued; and just as I was feeling more and
more relaxed and comfortable, I spotted Mort standing at the bar. I
quickly turned away to avoid his sighting me and told Tony I had to
leave. If Mort saw me he would expose me to the world. Mort was
unique in that he didn't care who knew he was gay, including his
parents. I admired his gutsy candor, but I wanted to "be someone"
someday—to have a wife, kids, career and respect. Being publicly
"out," Mort didn't have a snowball's chance in hell for any of
these. He lived for being gay, and was soon to lose his job and
begin his lifelong career as a gay bartender. This was not the life for
me.

Tony wanted to talk with me and suggested we go for coffee. I
agreed. Over the coffee he recounted his life and adventures as a
steward and as a homosexual. His stories of cosmopolitan trysts in
exotic cities fascinated me; but at the same time I felt his loneliness
as he hopped from city to city, body to body—countless bodies,
each used once, not in love, but in worship of the divine Orgasm. I
liked Tony, and it was a great relief to know that there were reasonably normal gay people in the world—as opposed to the twirly
queens lining the bar. I thanked Tony for the coffee and returned to
my tiny room at the Days Inn for a sleepless night of introspection. I
never saw him again.

The following morning I walked again down Hennepin Avenue—now strewn with beer bottles, vomit and trash from the night
before—towards the IDS tower, where I could catch the bus back to
school. As usual when I was early for the bus, I went into the IDS
tower's vast, glass-roofed, tree-filled atrium to sit and read the
newspaper. It was Sunday morning and the place was nearly deserted. Daydreaming, and watching the few tourists meander along
the concourse balcony above me, I saw a handsome blond man
leaning on the far balcony rail, taking in the atrium view. He was
quite a distance away, but I suspected he was looking at me. I went
back to my newspaper; when I looked up a couple of minutes later
he was gone. Soon I looked up again and he was on the balcony

immediately to my right. I averted my eyes from his stare, looked back, and again—gone. Minutes later there was a rustling noise from the bushes behind me. I turned and caught a glimpse of a face through the leaves. My imagination ran wild. Who was this mad stalker? Some FBI or CIA agent? What could he want from me?

Finally he emerged from behind the plant. He was about six foot two, with a perfectly chiseled face—a Cary Grant-like chin cleft complemented by high, broad cheekbones and deep-set, aqua eyes. As soon as we made eye contact, he flashed an almost ridiculously Ultrabrite smile. I smiled back. Well, then, it seemed introductions were in order. Scott Erikson was his name. He was a graphic illustrator, as evidenced by the two portfolios under his muscular arm. I asked if I could see his work, to which he replied, "Why not? But what do you have to show me in return?" In still-childish reflex, I lowered my head in embarrassment at this "I'll show you mine if you'll show me yours" invitation.

Although Scott's work consisted primarily of illustrating such exciting products as toilet bowl cleansers and laxatives, one could see that he did it with care, skill, and flair. He was 27 years old, and, coincidentally, had graduated from St. Olaf five years before. Most thrilling of all, he'd been captain of the football team. A jock, from my own school, now a professional, free, independent, and living in the city: What a package—and what inspiration for me! I asked what was in the other portfolio. "Just pictures," he replied. I insisted on seeing them. Seeming reluctant, he unzipped the portfolio. In addition to his graphic design work, he was a model. It was full of ads from Dayton's, Donaldson's, Marshall Fields, all featuring none other than Scott, page after fascinating page. But when I got near the end he pulled the portfolios away. I insisted on seeing the rest, grabbed it back and opened where I left off. It was a series of black and white nudes of himself which he had just picked up from his photographer. They (obviously) weren't for ads, nor were they porno; he had had them done simply for himself, and for the viewing pleasure of a few close friends who were undoubtedly as floored by his looks and physique as I was. To this day I have never seen such a beautiful body. Absolute, unrivalled Nordic perfection. On a scale from one to ten, Scott was a twelve.

He mentioned that as a boy he was heavy and uncoordinated, but puberty brought magical changes; a familiar story. I paid close heed as he explained how he was driven to better himself, and how small, daily improvements encouraged him to improve himself further. I had not yet achieved anything near his physical perfection, but for the first time I realized what I might become if I made the most of my raw materials. He would be my inspiration to develop my body.

He began looking me up and down, as though reading my mind, and said, "Jimmy, you will find throughout your life as a homosexual—if that is the life you choose—that having a hot body is of ultimate importance and will be one of the keys to happiness in your life."

I would never forget this remark. It haunted me throughout the remainder of my college career—indeed, throughout my life. While I would never match Scott, his words, and the living example of his body, inspired me to spend endless hours at the athletic center at school. I would never again be the butt of jokes and the target of towels. On the contrary, people would stare at me with admiration and envy. I would make sure of it.

Scott and I retired from the lush surroundings of the atrium to The Haberdashery, an English pub adjacent to the Radisson Hotel. We ordered drinks. Scott stared into my eyes with a mischievous gleam. Soon his muscular calf began to rub up and down against mine; then he planted his foot on my hardening crotch. I flushed with embarrassment. Scott saw how ill at ease I was carrying on this way in the bar, and invited me home to his apartment. He was everything I had dreamed of: a man's man; sexy, strong; this was an opportunity I could not pass up.

His flat was a full floor of an old brownstone tastefully done in a sort of minimalist Scandinavian style, appropriate for Minneapolis. The living room was dominated by a lifesize poster for the Chicago Film Festival, showing Scott with a beautiful woman wrapped around his torso. Scott was nude with the exception of a torn tank top through which his muscles bulged. Both bodies looked oiled and they glistened with beads of sweat as if they had just finished a session of wild sex. Their genitals were just hidden tantalizingly in the shadows. Noticing my admiration (drooling, practically), Scott went to his desk and pulled out a small print of the poster and autographed it, "To the sexy blond I'm going to show what it's all about." If I wasn't in love before, I was now.

As Scott and I undressed in his bedroom, I couldn't keep my eyes off him. The suggestive way he had unzipped his portfolio was a prelude to the way he now unzipped his pants. They dropped to the floor, exposing his thick, veined calves and well-rounded hamstrings — hairless except for light peach fuzz. The divinity in the poster was coming to life before my eyes. His great pendulum hung half-way down to his knees, and as I undressed, it grew even further. Though still flaccid, it was so large I imagined it would take a winch to get it up. The skin was smooth as velvet, covering only slightly the base of the head. Scott approached with tender eyes and with gentleness. We kissed long and hard, our tongues probing deeply. Between my legs I could feel him hardening. "Uh oh, my pookie's getting nasty," he purred, affecting the innocence of a five-year-old; nothing could have contrasted more with the sight of his flaccid member swelling into full, thick-veined, iron-hard erection. It was heavenly, but not easy, getting it into my mouth. We lay down in the 69 position and sucked each other for what seemed like hours, stopping only moments before our simultaneous explosions. I was in ecstasy. It had come to me at long last: the ultimate sexual experience with my male ideal; perfect in every sense — mind, body, personality, sensitivity, and above all, dick. Scott was, and remains, my ideal; every man I would meet thereafter would be measured against his monumental yardstick. Few have even come close.

I lay awake all night in his warm arms. All I could do was watch this beautiful man sleep. I left early next morning to try to catch the first bus back to Northfield for my Monday morning class. I missed it, but the night had been worth a week of missed classes.

I called Scott the next day and we arranged another meeting the following weekend. He came down to pick me up in his car on Friday afternoon (arriving about half an hour late, which made me a nervous wreck — didn't he want me anymore?). Before leaving St. Olaf, he wanted to look around his alma mater. As we drove around the campus, he reminisced about his days of athletic glory. When we reached the football field, Scott jumped over the door of his old Triumph Spitfire, ran to the goal post and actually hugged and kissed it as if it were a long lost love. I was both amused and moved by the display (although I could think of a post *I'd* have rather hugged and kissed).

We roared back to the Twin Cities, the sports car doing over 80. We stopped for burgers and fries, then proceeded home for the main course. We undressed simultaneously in a titillating, item-for-item striptease. When Scott had his pants down to his ankles, he stopped abruptly and threw me a shocking proposition: "Jimbo, have you ever had a dick up your ass?"

"Are you serious?" The idea of anything sexual concerning the anus or rectum was entirely new to me, and abhorrent. Scott insisted the experience was half of what "it" was all about. In and of itself, the idea seemed revolting; but with the sincerity in Scott's eyes, and his sheer beauty, I was ready and willing to try anything. Scott got some gel and massaged it up and down his penis.

"Lay down on your back," he told me. "Legs up on my shoulders."

As though hypnotized, I followed his orders. I would have followed him to hell and back at that point. He proceeded to finger my virgin asshole with the gel, preparing it for penetration as I shuddered with fear. Even after the joint we had smoked to relax, my rectal muscles tightened with every probe.

"Relax," he commanded. I tried. I wanted so badly to please him. Finally he pushed his dick head up against my hole; "Slowly, slowly," he murmured.

"No!" I yelped as the head of the huge shaft entered my hole. This went on for at least a half an hour. It was just not working. As a last resort, we retreated to mutual masturbation. I could sense Scott's disappointment. I wished I had been man enough to take it, but I was not ready mentally or physically. I was overcome with a feeling of inadequacy; I had failed him.

During the weeks that followed, I tried calling Scott repeatedly, only to get his answering machine. The recording was some sexy woman's voice couched in sleazy background music: "Sorry," she panted, "Scott can't come to the phone right now, he's . . . *busy.*" When I first heard it I was in hysterical laughter. After several times that turned into hysterics of a different kind; I wanted to rip the phone off the wall and strangle the woman with the cord. Now I knew how poor Blake Gallagher felt when Peggy and I did our little number on him at the Country Club. I never heard from Scott again.

My sophomore year was ending. I planned to take my usual summer job as a lifeguard, but went home to find the job had been given to another rich brat. My father, it turned out, was pleased. I was 19; the time to sever me from mommy's bosom, teach me the ropes of life, and develop my balls and guts, Dad felt, was long overdue. By this time he was Executive Vice-President at the Dubuque Packing Company. He used his pull to overrule the union contract and get me a job in the plant. My starting day came and I met him at his office. We walked together down a lonely corridor to the massive steel door of the plant itself. The mere sight of that door gave me a chill of foreboding; and indeed, despite its icy steel-blue color and the frigid air that lay beyond, it was to be my entrance to a summer of living hell.

The cutting foreman met me at the door and suggested I go by my first name only so as to obscure the fact that I was the boss's son and thus avoid union hassles. My first sight was of giant bloody pig carcasses traveling on huge steel hooks along a chained conveyor system, evoking nightmare visions of a concentration camp. Thirty or so men were above on a platform, each making his cut on the carcass. This was the season in which carcasses were often found to have been pregnant. From these, the amniotic sacs (along with various other guts) were removed, sent down a funnel and plopped into a large steel vat. My job would be to stand below the platform, pull the sacs, heavy and covered with blood and urine, out of the vat, cut the fetuses out and throw them into barrels of formaldehyde ice for shipment to laboratories where the bloodstreams would be latexed red or blue indicating arteries or veins. The fetuses would then be sent to biology departments of colleges and high schools for students to dissect.

The burly men in their bloodied smocks all looked up and stared as I walked in with the foreman and positioned myself for what was to be my nadir. The "cut" was explained to me and I was fitted with smock, gloves, boots and knife.

"Just dive in when you're ready, old Jimbo. Okay, Frank, start droppin' 'em."

Plop. Splat. As the first lower intestinal tract was dropped into the vat, I summoned up my own guts and plunged my hands into the mess, feeling the sickening warmth of the blood- and urine-covered entrails through my plastic-lined gloves. Once the initial horror passed, the process became routine. Communication with the rednecks was nil, with the exception of Lulu, an enormous mole-faced Pole, the only woman on the cut. The rednecks, with mouths as brutal as their brawn, faced with cleaning up their carnage at the end of the day, would usually dump the task on Lulu: "Get the Mole to do it, that's what women are for." Poor Lulu, a childless and husbandless woman, had been supporting herself and her bed-ridden mother from an early age. I would become like an adopted child and she, my protection from the other workers. Lulu was a gossip and would tell me about the others' private lives, most of which were disastrous stories of philandering, wife-beating and alcoholism.

I drove to work each day in Wimpy, a used Toyota station wagon I had bought from my mother and dad for $200 I'd earned by lawn mowing. Towards the middle of the summer, Wimpy broke down for three days and I had to make the trip to the Pack with my father in his big Lincoln Continental. Dad parked on the other side of the factory in front of the executive office entrance. Thus, the possibility of the workers seeing me was highly unlikely. The third morning, however, two workers from my cut walked by my father's office entrance as I jumped out of the car, looked at me and nodded their heads in recognition. I was discovered.

"Dad, they saw me."

"That's okay. Don't worry about it, Jimmy."

Later that day on the cut, a giant, bloody pig testicle came slamming into my head from out of nowhere. It felt like a football. Dazed, I looked up at the workers as they all played innocent. Soon after, the catcalls and name-calling began, not to mention an occasional push and shove in the lunchroom. I did my best to ignore it and with Lulu's help and friendship, I persevered; but the situation got worse. I pleaded with my father repeatedly for an office job; he refused. After all, this was my time for character strengthening and "balls" building. The climax of this misery was near the end of the summer when the pig fetus season was at its peak. As the flop of sacs became increasingly frequent (lending macabre new meaning to the expression "raining cats and dogs"), work became almost too grueling to keep up with.

One day as I was leaning over the vat to pull out an extraordinarily heavy sac filled with many fetuses, one of the workers above purposely kicked another bloody, uriny sac through the funnel. It fell on my head and dropped around my neck. This time the workers exploded into laughter as I gagged and ran puking to the steel door leading to my father's office.

"Dad, you told Mom when I was six that when I became 13 you wanted to take over and give me the balls and guts to deal with life. Well, I'm 19, and rest assured I've got them now, literally and figuratively."

He looked at me with a concurring and sympathetic smile. "Well, Jim, I guess you have."

I refused to return to my job. My summer of character building was over.

To preserve my sanity through this season of horror, I'd thought about the fall. I had to be compensated in *some* way for the gut and ball building I endured. I simply could not face the start of my junior year holed up in the stiflingly conservative world of rural St. Olaf. Now it was time to assess my alternatives. A semester of art history in Paris? Theater in London? Classical studies in Athens? Up to this point, my travels had included such exotic adventures as two weeks with my maternal grandparents in Florida, our fishing cabin in Perham, Minnesota, and of course, that whirlwind high school tour of Canada (and heterosexuality). The fall course catalogue came and my fingers raced immediately to foreign semester options. I wasn't particularly gifted or interested in any one field of study; but given my father's business orientation, I thought economics in London would sit well with him. I popped the question; he popped my balloon.

"Jimmy, world travel and material rewards are things you have to earn in life. You will do it someday on your own and will appreciate it much more that way. You'll look back and thank me for it."

"But Dad, haven't I earned something for my summer of living hell? I stuck it out, didn't I?"

"Yes, Jimmy, you did and I'm proud of you for it, but my word is final."

Crestfallen, I fumbled through the catalogue again and came across the Urban Studies program at Northwestern University in downtown Chicago. My father finally agreed to this compromise. The prospect of living in a big city excited me for innumerable reasons: the architecture, the stores, the political and society diversity . . . gay bars and gay men. No more pinball at the Oly bar scouting pussy and drinking till vomiting. I applied for the program, and in late August a letter came with instructions for orientation. It was to be held on September 6, 1977, the day before my twentieth birthday.

I had been to Chicago a few times, but only as a teenager, and only with my mother — although in a way, I engineered the trips myself. On weekends my mother would drive down to my father's office (in Dubuque) to call distant relatives on the WATS line. As a child I'd hated being dragged along; it meant her yakking for hours in Danish while I scoured vacant desks for gum and candy and played haunted house with myself on the upper floors. As it expanded in my early teens, the company bought an eight-seat prop jet. During one of my usual treasure hunts around the office, I found the log showing where the plane was scheduled to fly and whether there were extra seats available. If there were, we soon learned, my mother and I could tag along for a free ride, usually into Meigs Field in downtown Chicago for a day of shopping. From this discovery on, I would drive my mother crazy if she missed a weekend of calls, just so I could check the log. I lorded this perquisite over my classmates as if I were a character out of *Dynasty*. This, along with the ski area and my father's position, became my chief source of snobbery throughout my teens. People either hated my guts for it, or chummed up to me in hopes of getting in on a piece of the action. The latter, curiously enough, were the same ones who had tormented me for my obesity in years past. If my going to live in Chicago now galled them anew, so much the better.

Chapter 4

Iowa Boy in the Windy City

Vainglorious men are the scorn of the wise, the admiration of fools, the idols of paradise and the slaves of their own vanity.

—Jean-Paul Sartre

It was September 5 and the drive into Chicago seemed endless. I would have my reward after all. Twenty miles outside the city, the John Hancock Building and Sears Tower gleamed in the sunlight, like the proverbial pot of gold at the end of the rainbow after a summer storm. My excitement grew as we turned off the I-90 onto the Fulton Street exit in the Near North. "Here we are, Jim," Dad said. Mother sat chain-smoking and wringing her hands nervously as the time to give her son up to the city neared. (I couldn't wait.) The downtown campus of Northwestern was right on the lake, just north of the Loop. Finding parking space was next to impossible, which only compounded my impatience. We finally found a spot at the Administration Building entrance. They waited in the car as I ran in to get the key to my apartment, to which we proceeded.

The apartment was only three blocks west of campus, on the corner of State and Superior, kitty-corner from Holy Name Cathedral, seat of the Catholic diocese in Chicago. Just my luck: this would provide a constant reminder of the "damned if you do, saved if you don't" attitudes prevalent in my late, unlamented Dubuque. The massive limestone structure had copper doors that opened automatically as one approached; obviously meant to hint at the mysterious power of God, it in fact evoked nothing holier than a supermarket. ("Salvation? Aisle 2, on your left.") In any event, watching from my apartment window as unsuspecting churchgoers approached would prove only slightly less entertaining during my long, dull studies than the better bits of *Candid Camera*.

When my mother saw the apartment, she recoiled in something approaching horror. The building was one of the last remaining tenements in the area, the rest having yielded to skyscrapers and parking lots. The apartment was on the top floor of a six-floor walk-up, and helping carry up my belongings just about did my parents in. The living room and bedroom were in early hovel style. The kitchen was much livelier looking: it literally crawled with roaches. But, from the living room, a vintage iron spiral staircase rose to a second level where there was a huge room with bath and access to the rooftop. I was elated. My mother immediately got out pen and paper to write the program director to complain about the conditions they expected her son to live under. My father quietly took it in with a few chuckles, probably thinking it would contribute further to the building of my character.

When it was time to leave, my mother was in tears. My father merely extended a firm handshake and a "Good luck, Jimmy." By this point, what with their cigarette smoking and Mother's complaining, I felt I could bear to see them go. Besides, I was eager to go out to explore. Once semi-settled, I called information for the Gay Hotline. I figured if Minneapolis had one, Chicago was bound to. A fey voice answered and I asked the whereabouts of the nearest non-fey gay bar. "Alfie's on Rush Street, only blocks from you, dear. You'll love it. It's faaaaabulous!" . . . GAG!

It was Friday and I had the weekend in which to settle in. Later that day my roommates arrived: Tom, a jolly, fat Polish boy reeking of B.O. and cursed with a face pockmarked as a lunar landscape — the indelible record of an acne-afflicted adolescence; Guy, a wide-eyed Jewish Poindexter type from Skokie who carried Tolstoy and Dostoyevski around throughout the semester; and Ken, also Jewish, a rebellious type from a wealthy Winnetka family, with quasi-Afro hair and a guitar case plastered with women's lib, peace, anti-nuke and anti-everything-else stickers. Considering the purpose of the Urban Studies program — not career exploration so much as exposing a handful of sheltered, guilt-ridden rich kids to the wonderful world of social injustice — Ken was the perfect roommate. I would have been happy with Godzilla, as long as I had access to a social

life with (1) people liberal enough to deal with my sexual preference and (2) men who would (hopefully) fulfill my sexual needs.
On point one, my motley crew of roommates seemed okay. But
after a quick dinner with them at a cheap Chinese restaurant, I knew
they'd mean little more to me than someone to share the rent. My
social and sex life would, so to speak, lie elsewhere.

After a long morning of travel and an afternoon that was exhausting both physically (load after load up six flights) and emotionally
(dealing with the departure of my parents), the sagging, lumpy mattress offered quite sufficient invitation to slumberland. As my head
hit the musty pillow, my thoughts turned to Alfie's, where I'd decided to spend the following night, the eve of my twentieth birthday. The next day my usual birthday-period depression was miti-
gated by my excitement about the evening to come. With both a
cringe and a thrill that those days were behind me, I thought of the
birthdays of my past: the family, the sickening, white-frosted birthday cakes with sugary pink flowers, the fake smiles and forced
"thank you"'s and "beautiful"'s for new Sears catalogue underwear, tennis shoes, and double knit shirts. Tonight would be different, to say the least. Tonight would truly be *mine*.

I began the day lying on a towel on my rooftop, drinking in the
sun and the exhilarating skyline view. I would spend the day doing
everything possible to look and feel my best for my Chicago debut.
Late in the afternoon I started my workout: set after set of pull-ups
on an old clothes pole; biceps curls lifting plastic trash bags filled
with old telephone books found under the cockroach-infested
kitchen sink. The truly resourceful bodybuilder always finds a way.

As night neared, I checked myself out in the mirror one last time;
then another last time; about 30 or 40 "last times" in all. It was
only 9:30, and although the fey man on the hotline said "11" was
the best time for the bar, my patience was running out. My roommates had invited me to join them in some new adventure in culinary madness, but I'd politely declined. One final final glance in
the mirror and I was out on State Street and off to Alfie's. Childhood guilt-induced paranoia arose as I walked down the street. A
product of Sundown Town, only 3 1/2 hours away, I was terrified
of being found out. I pulled out my sunglasses as I approached the
bar (probably ensuring more attention than anonymity), kept walk-

ing briskly as if I were going to pass right by it, took a quick glance behind me, and literally jumped through the dark doorway. Sunglasses still on, I tripped on the doorman's foot and crashed into the wall.

"ID please," the doorman barked. I nervously fumbled through my wallet and produced my Iowa license, to which he responded, "Woo-wee, we got us a fresh young farm boy. He's gonna be a-squealin' like a pig a'fore ya know it." Great start. My big-city debut, and here I was some sort of hillbilly.

There were only three lonely men in the bar, two dressed in early Liberace, the third a beer-bellied, lonely-looking truck driver type who eyed me suspiciously. Excitement and anticipation instantly turned to depression and despair. Eleven o'clock, Jimmy, wait till then, I incanted as I downed one beer after another. Within an hour I was in a stupor and people were filling the club. As the music got going and I stumbled off the barstool, weaving through an unsavory-looking crowd, a sudden glimpse of three good-looking men who looked, even through the smoke and beer haze, absorbed in animated, sparkling conversation, brought me to attention. The middle one's eyes met mine, a smile curled up one side of his mouth, and his eyes narrowed. It was what I came to call, after I'd learned his name and his style, the trademark "Bud look." Bud was a tall, good-looking Rock Hudson type with cleft chin and thick, wavy brown hair who stood out like a swan amidst a gaggle of dirty pigeons. He wedged through the other two and approached with a "Hiya" that could sell swampland in Florida. We shook hands, and each went into a brief synopsis of our backgrounds. Bud Casey was born and raised in Blue Island, a lower-middle-class suburb on the South Side of Chicago, where he now worked in an uncle's costume jewelry store. He seemed totally devoid of pretense, which was a refreshing contrast to most gays' (myself included) constant striving to top each other socially, materially, and physically. I mentioned to Bud that it was my twentieth birthday; he responded with a smack on my cheek and congratulations at becoming an adult. We talked further as Bud sipped on his Bud and I on my Tanqueray and tonic, which was fast rendering me dizzy and sleepy. As handsome as I found him, I was too tired and my judgement too distorted to consider anything further. It was time to go.

We exchanged numbers and made plans for dinner early the following week.

I stumbled out of the bar and grabbed the southbound subway at Fulton Street, fell asleep, and woke up in the Loop on a train full of drunken gentlemen (speaking somewhat generously) staring in blank bewilderment at an equally dazed but totally out-of-place Iowa "farm boy." I decided to exit to a cab rather than wait for a northbound, for fear of muggers, stabbers, rapists, and other such forms of wildlife. I stumbled out of the cab back on State and Superior and struggled up the five flights to my hovel, in the process adorning the stairs with some of my beer and dinner. I fumbled with the keys for what seemed like hours, trying to open the triple lock which was, even under ideal conditions, akin to solving a Rubik's Cube. Once inside, I made my way up the spiral stairs in a clumsy but spirited race against my bladder. As I turned on the bathroom light, tiny clickety-clacks seemed to come from all over the room, and I just saw an army of cockroaches beating a hasty retreat into the walls. I must have screamed, because Ken sat up, startled, looking with his faux-Afro flattened on one side like a half-barbered Harpo Marx. My revulsion of the moment before instantly turned to hysterical laughter at this only somewhat less revolting sight. Ken yelled, "You goddamned drunken son of a bitch. You can take that pretentious alligator on your shirt and get fucked." But a moment later, we were *both* laughing hysterically. And from that time on, Ken and I were able to deal with our differences through laughter. I knew from day one that Ken was sensitive and intelligent. His outward scruffiness wasn't to my taste, but I recognized it as simply a rebellion against his wealthy, materialistic parents, and suspected he would get over it some day.

The next day Ken and I walked over to the Administration Building where we would embark on a week-long orientation to the city. Day One consisted of a subway ride to the poverty-stricken South Side for a tour of the projects and a visit to Jesse Jackson's Operation Push, an organization devoted to empowerment, headquartered in a crumbling Polish cathedral now transfigured by decay and graffiti. Inside, we were greeted — or *not* greeted, to be precise — by bulky black women desperately fanning themselves, and men in patent leather two-tone shoes, bright ties and polyester suits, shooting craps in a corner.

As our group entered, there was sudden silence and a sea of stares. Growing up in Sundown Town, my only two contacts with blacks had been at age five at O'Hare Airport with my mother, where I'd pointed a finger at an elderly black man and yelled, "Mommy, Mommy, why is that man's face so dirty?" (at which the man doubled up in laughter and my mother almost collapsed in embarrassment); and at age ten during a YMCA trip to Chicago, where at the Lincoln Park Zoo, a black man stole the applesauce cupcakes my mother had packed for my afternoon snack. So I'd have to admit that it was not without prejudice and apprehension that I now joined the hundred-odd black men and women in this church.

We took seats in the back and the service started. A choir, clothed in silver satin robes with hot pink sashes, launched into a jivey gospel tune and started swaying to and fro. On the second stanza the entire congregation joined in. The surge of emotion swept up everyone — myself included; the release was like nothing I'd ever experienced.

After the hymn, a roar arose as though Christ had returned and headed straight for the South Side (as I have no doubt he would). It was not Jesus, but Jesse — the Reverend Jackson. As he spoke or, rather, shouted, he was urged on by a steady chorus of "Uh huh"'s, "Lord have mercy"'s and "Amen"'s from the ecstatic crowd. The service ended with the gospel choir's rendition of "We Shall Overcome," after which everyone milled around exchanging smiles and greetings. This would be one of my very few memorable experiences from the Chicago Urban Studies program — although, on second thought, my *stomach* has never forgotten, nor forgiven, the Vietnamese restaurants, matzo ball fests, soup kitchens and soul food of some of our further adventures in ethnic subculture research.

I got home just in time to get a call from Bud.

"Movie? Dinner? Drinks?"

I was feeling game. "Well, how about all three?"

We agreed on 6:30. In only a week, my memory of Bud had faded behind that evening's drunken stupor. I vaguely remembered

Rock Hudson looks, but doubted I would recognize him on a street corner. Oddly, though, while I couldn't quite remember his looks, I could remember his *look* — the beguiling "Bud look." Anyway, it was a date.

Bud's apartment was in the Near North, in a standard U-shaped prewar building which seemed to be Chicago's version of the John Deere homes built for the factory workers in Dubuque — nondescript brick and nothing but the basics. With one knock, the door immediately swung open as if Bud were standing behind it waiting for me. The apartment consisted of a small room, closet, bath, and miniscule kitchen with dorm-sized refrigerator and two-burner stove. Bud told me to have a seat on the single bed, disguised for the daytime as a couch by overstuffed pillows. The place was decorated in Crate and Barrel Modern; reasonably tasteful — as good as could be expected on a Crate and Barrel budget. Bud went to the kitchen and returned with a bud vase containing a single red rose, which he placed on his drafting table-*cum*-dinner table. The meal consisted of salad, pasta primavera, and a lopsided homemade chocolate cake with big "2" and "0" birthday candles carefully placed in the middle. It was obvious that cooking was not Bud's forte, but the effort was sincere and, unbeknownst to me at the time, planted the seed which would only months later grow into a serious relationship.

Our second date was a bicycle ride along Lake Michigan and sunning at the Oak Street beach. As we stripped to our Speedos, I eagerly awaited the moment of truth, the supreme test, the ultimate question: Bud's body. (My, I'd become particular! Being an ex-fatso made me no more tolerant, no less exacting and demanding. Quite the contrary: It was as though I'd turned onto others the critical scrutiny *I'd* received for years.) Although no great shakes compared to Scott's physique, Bud's was acceptable, with a pleasing tuft of hair in the middle of the chest, a long, lean torso, and a trim waistline which, with a little work, had the promise of some muscular rippling. We spent the afternoon perusing the motley beach crowd, gawking at the bodybuilders' builds and ridiculing the rail-thin queens in shimmering lamé jock socks, swiveling their pathetic hips to and fro, the black ones screaming, "Girl" this and "Girl" that to each other, reminiscent of my Gay Nineties wig-snatching episode in Minneapolis. Bud's light Irish skin was soon turning red despite the sunscreen. Both of us looking forward to a first physical contact a bit more romantic than applying Noxema, we decided to pack it up for the day, and left the circus-like crowd to their antics.

At Bud's apartment we popped open beer cans and flipped a coin for the first shower. I won and, as seductively as possible, removed my togs. I languished in the shower beyond the squeaky-clean point, checking and double checking every crack and crevice for beach sand. I emerged from the shower and looked in the mirror, pleased with my renewed glow and tan lines. I applied after-sun lotion, tossed my hair into a perfect stylish wet look, and made my re-entrance. Bud was arranging things in his shoebox apartment, trying to lend it some atmosphere in preparation for the kill. As he stripped for his turn in the shower, I realized with disappointment where Bud got his nickname, as I spied what looked like a flesh-colored acorn peeking out from his crotch. But by the time of this shocking revelation, I was already lying on his bed, towel barely covering my privates (to make sure my bulge was obvious). I was committed — it would have been too awkward to back out. I liked Bud; our relationship had already gotten to the point where I couldn't hurt his feelings.

The sex — mutual sucking and masturbation — was devoid of passion; I had to think of Scott in order to maintain my erection. Bud, on the other hand, was lost in ecstasy. Immediately after we climaxed, he gave me his heart-rending Bud look. Despite my lack of sexual satisfaction, the look affected me enough to want to continue the relationship in some form.

Although Bud was 28, he was stuck in the rut of his lower-middle-class South Side roots. His days began with an hour and a half drive in rush-hour traffic to his uncle's Main Street jewelry store on the South Side. He would while away the hours behind a counter, selling zirconia brooches and fake pearls to glitz-loving blue-collar housewives. He had largely abandoned efforts to establish a career in graphic design and illustration, and focused instead on his social life. Secretly, I felt Bud's lack of success worked to my advantage: in my insecurity, I preferred to know he was as undirected and untalented as I; and, just as in my youth, I could feel socially superior based on my father's position. Bud served me best as nothing more than a handsome hunk; my personal ornament; a trophy. My sexual satisfaction, of course, would have to be obtained elsewhere. I continued to see Bud, but no more than once or twice a week; the rest of the time I spent out on the prowl looking for the ultimate sex machine, one whose physique matched Scott's, or topped it.

About six months into the relationship, Bud insisted I accompany him to a photography exhibit at the *Chicago Sun Times*. At the time, I had no interest in art per se, only perhaps in the status that knowledge of art could bestow. And even so, the only arts I was well versed in were my mother's kitschy crafts – découpage, macramé, tole painting, spice boards, and other such highbrow stuff. (You might say I didn't know much about art, but what I knew, I didn't like.) Nevertheless, I went along just to please Bud. He seemed unusually eager as we walked down the corridor to the exhibit. I couldn't wait to get through it and go sunbathing. Most of the photographs were fashion shots which I could have seen paging through *GQ*, *L'uomo*, *Vogue* or *Mademoiselle* at the supermarket. Then Bud stopped in front of a photo of a couple in trench coats strolling in the mist on the beach. "What do you think, Jim?"

"It's okay," I answered.

"Just okay?"

I looked again, then did a double or triple take. The man in the photo was Bud.

"How the hell did you get into that photo?" I barked.

"You'll see it in the paper tomorrow, Jimmy. It's an ad for Burberry. Isn't it great? My agent thought my look was 'it' for the job, sent my composite to Skrebneski and I got it." During the six months of our relationship, Bud had not uttered one word about modeling.

"Why didn't you tell me about this?"

"Didn't want anyone to think I was vain or conceited, especially if I failed."

Bud got the silent treatment the rest of the afternoon. I was consumed with jealousy. Just as the "Bud look" had planted the seed of our relationship, it now planted the seed of its destruction. And there it was in next day's paper: a half page that seemed to just scream "star quality." I instantly ripped it to shreds. My previous feelings for Bud – warm liking, complacency – were gone, transformed by the alchemy of jealousy into a corrosive mixture of intense love (or at least covetousness) and sheer hate. The photo was published internationally and instantly catapulted Bud into fame in the modeling world. People began approaching him with recognition and acclaim. Invitations of all sorts soon poured in; his agency fixed him up with beautiful escorts. He moved to the thirtieth floor of Sandburg Terrace, a Lincoln Park luxury highrise with a night view of the city as glittering as his new life. I stayed crammed into my Near North slum with my three stooges—Ken, Tom, and Guy.

Far from snubbing me, Bud tried to be nice. He was awkward, almost apologetic—as though he sensed my resentment and hurt. But his attempts to appease me only intensified my hatred. I was implacable, impossible. He would say green and I would say blue. His success had drilled deep down into me and tapped a dark, ugly reservoir, and the well was becoming a gusher.

Despite all this, with my first year at Northwestern ending, I made plans to return in the fall only to be with Bud; masochism, I suppose. As for the summer, my father, pleased with my meat packing efforts the year before, exercised his pull to get me hired at the Pack's boning plant on Chicago's Southwest Side.

The first day, I got into Wimpy—still with me, rustier, rattlier and more despised than ever—and headed off. It was still dark; work began at 6 a.m. I greeted Nick Parisi, head of the Chicago plant, in his opulent but tacky Las Vegas-style office. Nick sat puffing on his enormous Havana cigar behind a mammoth mahogany desk that only the heartiest of forklifts could have maneuvered. The floor was covered with orangish-brown, extra-deep shag carpeting—perhaps some sort of substitute for Nick's thinning hair. Nick affected a Bob Guccioni style: open shirt collar revealing a hairy chest and heavy, gaudy gold jewelry; an imposingly mafioso-like figure. He stood up, pulled his pants up over his protruding belly and boomed, "Jimmy, my boy, heard lots of good stuff about you from your dad. So now that you turned the Dubuque plant around, you want to give it a go here . . . yeah, good boy . . . 'course, ya come from good stock. Hardass, that old Kenny, but they don't come any better. C'mon, lemme introduce you to the Rabbi." This was Abe, a giant of a man, about 6 1/2 feet tall and about half as wide, with a nose that could have vacuumed Nick's carpeting. Abe personally slaughtered animals for kosher meat products.

"So dis is da kid wid da chutzpah? Ve'll put him to verk."

So far, to quote Yogi Berra, it was déjà vu all over again; I was back in last summer's multi-ethnic milieu. At least this time, the first name basis wasn't necessary, as "Melson" meant nothing to them. Anyway, I had almost no communication with the workers, not because of who *I* was but because the closest thing to English spoken was "South Side black."

This time my job was grabbing quarter fronts of beef with a thick iron hook and cutting the excess fat off with a machete-like knife. Because of the thickness and toughness of the material, I had to wear heavy cowhide gloves. Even so, within hours of the first day of hooking and chopping, my fingers were blistered and bloody.

"What time do we leave?" I asked Abe.

"Ven de quota's filled."

"What do you mean, when the quota's filled?"

"People gotta eat and if de markets don't have enough, ve have to stay and package more, until ve fill de orders. Sometimes ve leave at four-thirty, sometimes eight, nine o'clock. But ve like de overtime pay, time and a half."

"How about tonight?" I asked.

"Ven de horn blows, ve go, udervise ve keep verking."

My heart sank at the thought of not being able to make definite plans, and then, after a long, thrilling day with meat carcasses, crawling back exhausted to Bud, fresh from earning $250 for a two-hour shoot. After only the third day of work my hands were so swollen, my legs and arms so fatigued and my spirits so low, I couldn't go on. I walked into Nick's office and gave him the news.

"Nick, I did it one summer for my Dad, but enough is enough. The cut is a living hell and my heart aches for these people who do this day in and day out all their lives to support their wives and kids. But it's not for me. Not another summer. My college friends are working office jobs, traveling or waiting tables. I quit."

Nick pulled the cigar from his mouth, and instead of the barrage of obscenities I'd expected, said, "It's okay, Jimmy, I don't blame you; it's a damned tough job. We'll think of something to tell your dad. I'll tell him it's the racial thing. Now, go on, get outta here."

He offered his bear paw. "Good luck to ya, kid." I left his office feeling like a prisoner freed from Alcatraz.

As Wimpy and I made our way back to the Near North, I thought about other summer jobs. I had definitely had my fill of factory jobs, but had never worked in an office, nor bussed, nor waitered. I was well past the babysitting stage, and the thought of returning to another summer in Sundown Town and being without Bud was frighteningly depressing. Waiting tables seemed the best plan.

As soon as I got home I showered, scrubbing away as if to remove any hint, indeed even the memory of the accursed charnel house. I then primped and preened as if going on a first date, while concocting a mental résumé of my restaurant experience. I had lied all my life about my sexuality, so why wouldn't this work as well?

One last, long glance in the mirror (well, love is love) and I was out the door. I took State up to Rush, the hub of Chicago's eateries and nightclubs. After a few "Sorry, we're staffed for the summers", I stopped at Café de Harvey's, a trendy alfresco restaurant by day and club by night, and was directed to the manager's office by an androgynous waiter who vamped, "Careful, he'll maul you." My nerves still ragged from confronting big Nick, this was the last thing I wanted to hear. But what the hell, I thought, what do I have to lose?

I knocked, and a courage-shriveling "Waddaya want?" blasted from behind the door.

"Just looking for a waiter's job, sir. My name's Jim Melson." The door swung open to a chubby, mustachioed, mid-fortyish man who was a dead ringer for Rip Taylor. His hair was orangish — obviously a failed attempt at blond; vast quantities of hair spray kept it nice and hard, in a style that would have been the envy of Duane's Villa de Coiffure of Dubuque.

"So tell me, Mr. Whatchamacallit, what makes you think you can serve the brutal crowd that frequents my famous, or dare I say, infamous establishment? You look like a greenhorn just graduated from Lake Forest Academy. Probably a homecoming queen at that. You've probably never served food to fish, much less people. I'll tell you what, I just fired a wimp I caught drinking on his shift. I'll give you a try. You've got a cute tush, which should get people in off the street. Start tomorrow, 10 a.m. My name is Harvey Garland.

However, you will call me Mr. Garland. Only my friends receive the privilege of calling me Harv. Now, if you will kindly remove yourself from this office, I am a very busy man."

"Thank you, Mr. Garland; you won't regret it. I really appreciate. . . ."

"Did you hear me, Mr. Melson?"

"Yes, sir." I was elated. I would surely be seen and discovered as Bud had been.

On my way out, I ran into the waiter who had directed me in. "I overheard your conversation with Harv — congratulations. Just know one thing: Those who call Harv 'Harv' are those who *have*." He paused to let his meaning sink in. "He's 'Mr. Garland' to those who *haven't*. And those who *won't* probably won't be here long." Needless to say, Mr. Garland could remain Mr. Garland as far as I was concerned.

The following day, Bud prepared a special culinary effort for dinner, for which I carefully planned a display of extreme distaste. Bud seemed strangely uptight throughout the meal; absent was his usual joviality. At the end, he looked at me intently.

"Jimmy, there's something I want to tell you. This has been coming for a long time and I want you to know how special you are . . . but I . . ."

"Just get to the point."

"Okay, I just don't think I love you anymore."

"Oh, come on, Bud, give me a break, you've always been whipped on me. Big joke."

"Jimmy, I'm serious. Ever since the Skrebneski shot, it's been a downhill slide. We're different people now, leading different lives. You've been doing this guilt trip number on me and I'm at wit's end to please. I just can't deal with your jealousy anymore. It's over. Just remember, you are very special. You'll be a star someday. You don't want to tag along on my coattails. You want the limelight and you deserve it."

"I don't believe you. I don't fucking believe you. Here I've changed my life around with school and work just so I could be with you, and this is my reward? Excuse me, I have to use the bathroom." On the wall above the towel rack was a glass-framed silkscreen of James Taylor I'd given Bud as a memento of our relationship. I ripped the picture off the wall and flung it against the medicine cabinet mirror, producing an explosion of shattered glass. Bud screamed and pounded on the door.

"What the hell are you doing?"

"Oh, just destroying any reminders of me before you do. If you want, I'll return the tape you gave me." (Also James Taylor. Who needed to hear the lyrics, " Whenever I see your smiling face, I have to smile myself," now that the true sentiment was "Whenever I see your frowning face, I have to say fuck off"?)

"I hate you, hate you, hate you," I ranted. "How could you do this? You've probably fallen in love with yourself. Mirror, mirror on the door, look at Bud, what a bore. Mirror, mirror on the wall, see Bud's dick, isn't it small?"

My rising temper was attaining lyrical heights. ("O for a muse of fire" indeed.) Bud's lower jaw jutted forward, teeth clenched; he continued to stare in silence as I ranted and raved — and so too when my raving gave way to pleading and begging for reconsideration. Finally, in despair, I demanded he take me to the airport so I could fly home.

"Sure, Jim. Can I help you pack?"

"No, I can do it myself. I don't want you touching my stuff. Just pick me up in one hour." As I slammed the door, I slumped to the floor in wailing sobs, hoping Bud would hear, open the door and relent. I had no idea where I was going to go, but knew I had to get out of Chicago. Despite the opportunity *chez* Garland, I knew I couldn't bear being in a city plastered everywhere with Bud's face. Mr. Garland would have to find his new "Harv" prospects elsewhere. I would show Bud somehow. Someday he would regret this moment.

Bud was silent as he drove the I-90 to O'Hare on that gray day. I kept checking his face for some sign of emotion but there was none; he just stared straight ahead. We pulled up to American Airlines and I hauled my baggage out of the trunk, then looked in the passenger window with a kicked-puppy-dog look. "Are you sure, Bud? I have lived for you and through you. I don't think I can go on. You are my life."

"But that's the root of the problem, Jimmy. I'm 29 and have finally made a dent in this world. You're only 20. Your time will come, and besides, you aren't in love with me, you're in love with the image. Best of luck and keep in touch once in a while, okay?''

I shut the door and watched helplessly as Bud drove off into the gray distance. Where was I going to go? I didn't even have reservations. Mom and Dad certainly weren't expecting me and I was emphatic about not returning to Dubuque for the summer. I picked up a discarded *Tribune*, mindlessly turning through the pages to relieve my trauma, and there was Bud — not once but twice — teeth, dimples, chin cleft and all. I ripped the *Tribune* to shreds. An old lady sitting nearby chirped, "Good heavens, dear, what's the matter? Are you alright?''

"It's just the trash they publish these days. I think its disgusting.'' I ran tearfully to make a desperation call to Gabe Reynolds, a friend of Bud's and mine. Gabe was a WASPy black who worked in production on ABC Sports. He attached himself to the modeling set like a tick on a greyhound looking to go along for the ride. In his horn-rimmed glasses, Lacoste shirt and Polo cords, he looked a bit like Bryant Gumbel. The ubiquitous Gabe showed up solo at the choicest society dinners, fashion shows and galas extraordinaire boasting about his life with the broadcasting set — Tom Brokaw, Cheryl Tiegs, Jane Pauley. Who knew if any of it was true? Well, no one could prove it wasn't. He was a total enigma, but always entertaining, and dependable for consolation.

"Gabe, this is Jimmy. I'm at O'Hare. Bud just dumped me and I'm a mess. What the hell am I going to do? I can't handle Northwestern this fall, much less Chicago, constantly hearing 'did you see Bud in?,' 'he looks great in,' 'how are you and that sexy model doing?' etcetera, etcetera, et fucking cetera. Not to mention seeing him plastered in every publication I pick up.''

"Jimmy, you knew this was going to happen. Everyone could see it coming. I have an idea. It's just an idea. Remember me telling you about my friend Spencer from New York? Old New York family? Cape Cod house? Park Avenue apartment? Forrest furniture? Loves blonds? Just listen. Go to New York. I'll call Spencer and see if he'll put you up for a few days. Get Bud out of your system and have a ball. New York makes Chicago look like Podunk. Let me call him right now. Give me your number, stay put and I'll call you right back. Trust mother.'' If I trusted mother, my nose would be buried in the books on Manitou Heights. Within ten minutes the phone rang.

"Gabe?"

"Jimmy, this is Spencer. Love to put you up. Why don't you just hop on the next flight out? My address is 970 Park Avenue. I've got a roommate, but he won't care and there's a guest room and study where you'll have plenty of privacy to do whatever.

Park Avenue! "Newww York is where I'd rather stay!" I almost sang out, à la Eva Gabor in the immortal balcony scene from *Green Acres*. "I get allergic smelling hay!" Yeah! Take country life and *shove it*, Eddie "Olivah" Albert! "I just adore a penthouse view, Dahling I love you but give me Park Avenue!"

I quickly recomposed myself. "Are you sure, Spencer? I couldn't impose on you like this. It's so spur-of-the-moment . . . but tempting as hell. . . . see you for dinner?"

"Great! Give me a call when you get in."

Piled on top of the pain of losing Bud, I now had excitement about New York, plus a rich topping of confusion. Result: emotional indigestion. What would I be getting into? What might I lose? In the end, adventure prevailed over caution. There was nothing written in stone that said one had to graduate from college in just four years. The lure of a Park Avenue invitation was simply too hard to pass up. My heart had been broken twice—first Scott, now Bud. I would show them both. I would become the heartbreaker, no longer the heartbreakee.

Knowing my mother would have a conniption fit if she knew about my little venture, I kept quiet. There was no reason to let her know.

Chapter 5

"New York Is Where I'd Rather Stay"

There is nothing to which men cling more tenaciously than the privileges of class.

—Leonard Sidney Woolf

Throughout the flight to New York, Gabe's remark that compared to New York, Chicago looked like Podunk kept ringing in my ears. If this was true, how could I ever return? Would I become lost in a world of lust and glamour? I certainly hoped so. Would Bud stew in his own juice upon seeing me in the pages of the *National Enquirer*, *People*, and *Interview*, hobnobbing with celebrities extraordinaire? Would I be hounded by paparazzi as I hopped in and out of limos from premieres to galas to clubs? Even while fantasizing, I bore in mind Gabe's reputation for exaggerating about his fabulous friends and connections. On the other hand, Spencer sounded for real, at least on the phone. Gabe apparently *could* cultivate some really impressive, friends.

As we approached and then circled Manhattan, a galaxy of lights from horizon to mind-boggling horizon spread itself below me like some fabulous carpet, as though to affirm my delirious New York fantasies. But I soon came back down to earth, both literally and figuratively, as I found myself amid a maddening airport mob of raw-nerved New Yorkers in full Friday-night flight to escape the city. Why so many seemed so eager to escape what I was so eager to enter, I could not (yet) fathom. I could only thank my lucky stars that I traveled opposite the bumper-to-bumper traffic. The bug-eyed cab driver made the run to the city in Grand-Prix style, and within minutes a line of sparkling skyscrapers came into view, so ab-

surdly, almost self-consciously theatrical — like the sequined stars
of some Broadway show on metropolitan scale, lined up for their
curtain call — I almost broke into applause. Easy enough to guess
what song was running through my mind; if I could make it here, I
could make it anywhere — but *would* I make it here, or disappear
among the millions, as mediocre as I'd always been, only more
anonymous?

My father's fascination with lurid Cagneyesque crime dramas
must have rubbed off on me, for as we drove through the Queens-
Midtown Tunnel under the East River, I thought of the remains of
Mafia victims in the mud above — skeletons chained to cement-
block "gravestones." I told the cabby to drop me off at P. J.
Clark's where I was to meet Spencer for drinks and dinner. Spencer
wanted to spare me the scrutiny of his nosy, highhanded doorman
who, if I arrived alone, would doubtless challenge my right to come
anywhere near his castle. "Doormen are worse than women under
hair dryers, Jimmy," Spencer had added when I called from the
airport. "They thrive on gossip. There are rumors that this building
is going co-op. If so, I don't want to blow my chances before some
snooty board. It's enough to have to tip them five every time they
open a cab door, without having to pay them off to keep their
mouths shut about the comings and goings of my guests."

P. J. Clark's was a historic landmark, a lone small brick building
standing defiantly amid the giant glass boxes of Third Avenue in the
East Fifties; its clientele had been loyal and influential enough to
save it from the development juggernaut. Thoroughly humble from
the outside, it was the interior that showed why it bore such senti-
mental value: It was as if a tornado had lifted up an English country
pub and plunked it down à la Wizard of Oz in midtown Manhattan;
truly an oasis from the maddening traffic outside. The crowd
seemed to be a mix of regulars and celebrity seekers, the latter
drawn by frequent mentions in the gossip columns of appearances
by Jackie O.

I had arrived well ahead of my meeting time with Spencer
(thanks to my cabby's Indy-style driving), so I downed a couple of
beers to calm my nerves. Alas, I had inherited my mother's pea-size
bladder (my life to date seemed like a constant search for public
places of relief). I was soon in the men's room, peeing into one of

the ancient, cracked urinals. As I was giving it the final shake, I noticed the man at the next relief station—a curly-haired, Anglo-looking man in kelly green Brooks cords, button-down shirt and Topsiders—eyeing me from head to toe and lingering somewhere in between. I had detested the idea of bathroom sex ever since hearing about Mort's sleazy debut at the Julien Hotel. There was a reason, in my opinion, why bathrooms and bedrooms were separated by a thing called a wall. I turned towards him as I zipped up my pants, about to call him a pervert, when he chirped, "Jimmy?"

"Spencer?"

"Well, welcome to the city of surprises!" And he burst into laughter.

We went and sat down. "We'll do our best to get your mind off this thing you call Bud," Spencer said. "Gabe tells me you're a Dane; you should really appreciate the smorgasbord of men this city has to offer." True enough, I was eager to sample every tasty morsel.

After a quick burger we cabbed up majestic Park Avenue to Spencer's elegant prewar building, where doormen in captain's hats and brass-buttoned, double-breasted dark green uniforms with epaulets greeted us with military briskness: "Good evening, Mr. Forrest." The cab door was opened for us and the baggage literally grabbed from my hands. Spencer stuffed a five in the concierge's hand while sending me a mock-world-weary look that said "does it ever end?" As we walked down the red-carpeted path through the Chippendale-filled lobby to the elevator, the full import of "Dahling I love you but give me Park Avenue" was abundantly clear. (What wisdom is not to be found in *Green Acres?*) It was, to say the least, overwhelming to a bumpkin from Iowa who had as yet experienced nothing more elegant than the Dubuque Golf and Country Club. The elevator opened on eight to an ornate gilt- and gesso-encrusted mirror which hung over an inlaid-marble-topped bombé chest. Here I was, a guest at one of the crème de la crème of New York addresses, if not the world, wishing only that I could shove this coup in Bud's face—not to mention those of all my childhood tormentors—to make my triumph complete.

Spencer directed me to my room in back of the kitchen, in former servants' quarters now converted to a self-sufficient guest apartment. After unpacking, I was to meet Spencer in his living room for a glass of vintage port and a soothing serenade of Rogers and Hart on an antique Steinway grand piano, Spencer's prize possession. Though he now ran the New York showroom of his family's furniture company, Spencer had studied music at Trinity College in England and was an accomplished organist who performed at St. Mary of the Virgin ("Smokey Mary's"), one of Manhattan's grandest Episcopal churches. For all that Gabe's wondrous stories were worth, Spencer could easily have turned out to be some aging queen in a garishly furnished coldwater flat. But here, sure enough, was the epitome of an old-guard, East Coast WASP, with looks, manners and understated style redolent of generations of upper class breeding. As one would expect, he took his money for granted, as almost a God-given birthright; unlike most gays I'd met, who didn't have two dimes to rub together yet flaunted Gucci wallets and Louis Vuitton luggage financed by overdrawn checking accounts, Spencer didn't need to prove himself to anyone. Totally unaffected and self-assured, he could easily have been mistaken for a first cousin of Prince Charles. I may not have been what you'd call worldly, but my judgement of character was already highly developed by hard lessons at the hands of people who abused me as a child and used me as an adult. My mother had always espoused a "never judge a book by its cover" philosophy, but she was wrong. The cover was an expression of the text; outward simplicity usually betokened honesty, humility and integrity; affectation signaled superficiality, greed and vanity. Spencer clearly possessed the grace and ease that only old money could foster.

All this breeding and style and refinement and wealth etc., etc., notwithstanding, a couple of Tanqueray and tonics soon revealed another side of Spencer: an incredibly campy sense of humor. Most of this was of the prep-school-homosexual variety, with an admixture of summer-camp naughty-boy experiences, and an overlay of drily sophisticated Episcopalian-brotherhood organist-guild wit. His routine included draglike send-ups of the Queen Mother, Julia Child and Barbara Cartland. I had assumed that with their robes, vestments, incense and bishops' mitre hats, Episcopalians were no more than a high-class version of Dubuque Catholics, with the same "If you're gay or eat meat on Friday you're damned to hell" attitude. I discovered that despite their Anglican, high-church origins, Episcopalians were very liberal with regard to race, sexual preference, abortion and so forth. Indeed, a goodly portion of the brotherhood were homosexuals. Meeting Spencer would ultimately lead me to join their church.

Next morning Spencer handed me a set of keys as he left for Forrest Furniture's High Point, North Carolina office. "I'm sorry I can't give you the royal tour, Jimmy, but business calls. I'll be gone for three days, so you're on your own. I just want you to be comfortable and consider my home yours. You can trash the place all you want, except for the piano; it almost dates back to old Ludwig himself. And don't let a pudgy black face staring at you on Friday morning startle you, its only Carlotta, the maid. Her name is quite appropriate; there's a *lotta* Carlotta. But she's a sweetheart." As soon as Spencer left, I roamed the apartment imagining it were mine, caressing the Chippendale dinner seating for ten, admiring the silver-framed photos (Spencer's family summering at the Cape, Spencer with classmates from Choate, his prep school, Spencer in Europe) and performing "Chopsticks" on the grand with all the coordination of a palsy victim.

The only place I wanted to be even more than inside this apartment was outside, seeing Manhattan. I decided I would first venture over to Broadway and Times Square—the theater district, the lights, the action, and, corny though it was, the place where the ball dropped on New Year's Eve that I used to beg my parents to let me stay up and watch on TV.

Downstairs, after the doorman opened the door, tipped his hat and hailed a cab for me, I reached into my pockets to tip him but found only fifteen cents. My wallet held a fifty dollar bill and traveler's checks, so fifteen cents it was. From then on, the hat stayed on and cab hailing and door opening was up to me. The cab dropped me at 42nd and Broadway. Although teeming with elegant theater goers at night, by day the area harbored nothing but bag ladies, drug dealers and hustlers, intermingled with a few fat Midwestern tourists reminding me painfully of what I wanted to forget. Times Square was nothing but a small garbage-littered triangle. On Fifth Avenue, where I went to gawk at New York's finest stores, angry cab drivers honked their horns at the double-parked limousines waiting for their wealthy matrons to emerge laden with jewels and clothes — the spoils of marriages to Wall Street brokers and lawyers, marriages with a more than superficial resemblance to high-class prostitution. As for men, the delicious "smorgasbord" Spencer had alluded to seemed, so far, more like spoiled leftovers unfit to feed stray cats.

After this disappointing introduction to Manhattan, I sheepishly reentered the lobby of 970 Park, making a quick beeline for the elevator — avoiding eye contact with the undertipped and undergrateful doorman. Back in the lap of Spencer's luxury, I removed my mustard- and ketchup-stained clothes, reeking of roasted chestnuts and New York pollution, and prepared a scented bubble bath in the mammoth tub. Then I searched Spencer's vast classical music library for just the right symphony, and his liquor cabinet for just the right fine liqueur. Mozart and cognac: a formula guaranteed to purge my soul of any remaining Midwestern hokeyness and imbue it with worldliness and culture. I admit this didn't come close to the high life of Dubuque — to wallowing in pig blood and guts, then coming home to case after case of Pickett's beer, Dubuque's home-made finest, growing fat in crushed velvet Barca-lounge chairs, watching pro wrestling, *Laugh-In* and *All in the Family*. Still, it was nice in its own way.

After a half hour of reveling in bubbles and glorious music I dried off and donned my robin's egg blue mini briefs, thrift shop vest, tuxedo shirt and coveted Frye boots, the couture de rigueur of the collegiate prep. With ravenous pot-induced munchies, I headed south to P. J. Clark's, hell-bent on bleu cheese burgers and cottage fries. A couple of extra pounds on me wouldn't drive away any supercharged studs. But once in the restaurant, the better angels of my nature, or at least my physique, piped up: "Don't do it, Jimmy! You've achieved as close as you can to physical perfection; keep it. Yield not unto temptation. You've won this battle; don't snatch defeat from the jaws of victory. Keep *your* jaws shut."

And so I soon heard myself mumble glumly to the waiter, "Spinach salad, please."

"You don't look like the type that a 'ladies who lunch' meal would satisfy for dinner . . . why don't you get the prime rib? It's inches thick and USDA prime choice."

"Sorry, I grew up on that stuff and it turned me into a prime porker. I don't want to go through that again."

"Ah, go for it. You'll burn it off dancing in the clubs. And as an objective observer, you look like a prime cut yourself." Well. I didn't have to be hit over the head to get his message. I didn't need ESP to catch his drift. He didn't have to draw me a picture. I *got* the picture. This guy had, shall we say, an appreciation for men. And being a bartender, maybe he could clue me in on the New York hot spots.

"Oh, speaking of clubs, I'm new in town—what do you recommend?"

"Shit man, head over to 54; it's the best fuckin' disco in the world."

"I'm sure it is. All you have to do is pick up *People* or the *Enquirer* to see all the celebrities who go there. But I couldn't get in; I'm not famous, nor am I blessed with a trust fund. Look at me; half my clothes are thrift shop."

"Listen, just look like you own the place at the door and you'll have no problem. You look perfect."

After paying my check (and tipping the bartender extra for his tip), I grabbed a cab to West 54th Street to find a mob scene on the street below the illuminated 54 sign. Limos were double-parked and more kept arriving. The doorman handpicked those lucky enough to gain attention and, like a Moses with blond hair and shades, parted the crowd like a human Red Sea to allow the Chosen People to enter. This doorman (Mark Beneke, as I later learned) made selection into a science. No democracy, this; a pure dictatorship of beauty, fame, style, wealth, power—or outrageousness. I had inched my way toward the black velvet rope, and was horrified to see Beneke toss a drink in the face of a gold-chained New Jersey type attempting to impress his overly made-up sex kitten date by offering a $20 bribe. The man lunged toward Beneke only to be confronted by hundreds of pounds of muscled bouncers; he had as much chance as a kindergartener up against the New York Giants defensive line. His girlfriend, who had undoubtedly spent hours, not to mention half a week's pay, on dressing for her metamorphosis from secretary to disco debutante, seethed in embarrassment and frustration and shrieked obscenities at Beneke. He just threw his head back and laughed, reveling in his power trip: "Back to 42nd Street, douche bag." Just as I was about to withdraw to avoid becoming Beneke's next victim, he pointed his finger over the crowd, motioning me forward. I looked back, expecting to see some celebrity emerging from a limousine, but there was none.

"How many?"

"How many what?"

"How many in your party?"

"Oh, uh, just me. I'm meeting friends."

"No charge for this one, Tony." I couldn't believe it, I was actually one of the Chosen! It *couldn't* be because I had the right Studio stuff; I assumed that Beneke figured if he treated *every* nobody in the same manner, as he had the previous would-be's, the crowds outside would soon disappear, followed by the club itself.

Following me in was Margaux Hemingway (unmistakable with those eyebrows) and her entourage. As the guards clipped the velvet rope shut, the crowd surged forward, calling "Mark, me, me, please, come on, come on!!!" I strutted through the smokey mirrored corridor to the pounding beat of Donna Summer as if I *did* own the place. Past the coat check was a diamond-shaped bar tended by flawless bare-chested and bowtied men pouring drinks at a speed that only a gram of coke each could have sustained. Precursors of the Chippendale's dancers, their sweaty torsos reminded me of Scott's, and their lascivious swaying and grinding to the music had patrons drooling on the bar and throwing bills their way.

Studio 54 was a converted grand old Broadway theater in which a dance floor and state-of-the-art sound and lighting systems had been installed. As the music would peak, hundreds of balloons and masses of confetti would cascade from the proscenium heights, and a quarter-moon face would swing down from the ceiling and "snort" a giant spoonful of coke, in celebratory imitation of most of the patrons' own doings. Once you *did* gain entrée to the club, the atmosphere was devoid of the pretenses, the "attitude," that prevailed among those left standing outside. Everyone could let his hair down; royalty would dance with rock stars, Eurotrash with debutantes, and pro athletes with the likes of Disco Sally and Rollerena, two of the notables of the "outrageous" category. Disco Sally was a 4 1/2-foot-tall woman in her mid-seventies who usually ended up in the middle of the dance floor on the shoulders of some bare-torsoed musclebound stud, an ethyl-chloride-soaked rag stuffed in her mouth, arms flailing wildly with the beat; in short, much like your grandmother or mine. Rollerena was your typical stockbroker-by-day, drag-queen-by-night, wearing exactly what one would expect — owlish spectacles, antique wedding gown, and roller skates. S/he would pass wordless and expressionless through the crowd with wand in hand, pause to give this or that disco prince or princess a tap of approval and then move on. Only the most discreet of the paparazzi were allowed into the club, as the wrong kind of public tabloid exposure could ruin careers and reputations (which needless to say, could also benefit incalculably from — indeed, depend entirely on — the right kind).

My first eye-to-eye contact was with a man with blondish red hair, wearing a Cardin tuxedo and shmoozing with Nan Kempner, Truman Capote, Gloria Vanderbilt and some others. He spotted me and nodded subtly toward a vacant banquette without his companions noticing. Why not? I thought. I had to start somewhere, and from his looks and his stellar acquaintances, he seemed the ideal candidate to introduce me to the best the city had to offer. He excused himself from his group with a European-style kiss on both cheeks of each of them, men included. That little gesture impressed me; the urbanity, the sophistication of it — *and* the certain knowledge that it would make most Dubuquers recoil in disgust and retreat to the moral propriety of their Elks Clubs and Masonic Lodges.

He snapped his fingers at one of the macho waiters, ordered Chivas for two, joined me at the banquette, and introduced himself as Walter Montfort. "Heavens, child," he effused, "you are a divine creature . . . obviously unspoiled and untainted by all this delicious corruption. Tell me about yourself. You have the whole group agog. Let me take a guess. You could be a model, but your looks suggest that there's something more to you than that airheaded narcissistic bullshit. Your cowboy boots indicate you're not of the East Coast prep breed, and your clothes aren't trendy or beachy enough to suggest California. I got it. I got it. You are a corn- and cattle-fed Midwesterner, sick and tired of farm country,

and lured here by the bright lights and high times you've read about
in *People* magazine.''

Stunned and slightly wounded by his uncanny perception, almost
without thinking I concocted a face-saver: ''Actually, I'm here doing a study for my thesis comparing the decline of American civilization to the fall of the Roman Empire.''

''Quick thinking. What's your methodology? Observational or
participatory?''

''Oh, a bit of both, I think.''

''Well, good to hear, love, because if your intentions are strictly
observational, better get yourself a chastity belt and prepare for a
poor grade. But if they're participatory, fasten your seatbelt, join
the party and experience the decline of American civilization first
hand. You'll love it. It's addicting. I'm offering my services as
your personal escort so you can observe *and* participate in the best
that decadence has to offer. Here, try a toot. Hundred dollars a
gram. It's the best! Rubell makes sure that the most desirable of his
clients are well taken care of so they keep coming back. That's what
creates the mystique of this place. It's all in the basement. Come
on, I'll give you the celebrity tour.''

He grabbed my hand and led me to an inconspicuous, flat-black-
painted door and down creaky stairs into Studio's notorious basement. In bizarre contrast to the boiler room setting, small groups of
noted celebs sat around on thrift shop furniture receiving chemical
''party favors.'' Everywhere were tabloid-familiar faces. Noticing
me standing alone awkwardly while Walter circulated, greeting the
regular basement luminaries, the Princess Diane Von Furstenberg
approached me and oozed, Garbo-fashion, ''Dahling, velcome to
ze basement. Alzough it looks like hell, really it's heaven. Come,
sit viz me.'' She grabbed my hand, pulled me onto her lap, and
stuck her tongue into my ear. At just about that moment my first
toot of coke kicked in, lending the grubby basement, and its occu-
pants, brilliance and grandeur. It truly did seem like an underground heaven.

''You're perfect, Diane,'' I purred idiotically.

''No, you're perfect. Everyone here is perfect. This place is perfect.'' On and on went this exercise in tag-team narcissism, this
coke-driven *folie à deux*, both of us hearing profound insight in

every word. Someone could have spit on me, and that would have been "perfect" too. Everyone floated around in this "I know you, you know me, we're all beautiful" love-in a while longer; then the muffled beat of music upstairs began to beckon, drawing us up like a Hindu's cobra (for were not we, too, well-charged with "poison"?). We flirted, sweated and ground to the rhythm until the early morning; then the lights dimmed; it was time for the show. With a lengthy, pulsating prelude, the DJ teased the audience into a near-riot level of excitement. Smoke guns filled the stage floor with white mist, the ether of mystery into which the disco diva now made her ethereal entrance. A black, specterlike figure slowly materialized, and the deep, exotic vibrato filled the room: Eartha Kitt singing "I Need a Man."

By a couple of hours later, the show had ended; the music had shifted from fifth gear back to third, the last champagne corks had long since been popped, the best of the coke had been snorted, the best of the models had departed in anticipation of next day's shooting. Left were only the most undisciplined ones, lost in self-abandon and headed for self-destruction. (Plus, of course, your faithful "observer" of civilization's decline.) These stumbled at last down the long dark corridor to exit into the shocking morning sun. These were the disco dilettantes — here one day and gone the next — who spent what money they had on drugs and always woke up next afternoon depleted, depressed — and already thinking about how to pay for their next blowout. Sooner or later they found themselves on a Greyhound back to Ohio, or their looks ravaged by their excesses, no longer able to attract Beneke's eye and gain entrée.

The following morning I awoke, startled, to find a gorgeous Italian-looking guy snoring beside me. And what had woken me was the sound of someone closing the door to my room. Oh, my God. Spencer's maid — I forgot. Although the snorer was truly a Donatello, I poked him and informed him that his departure was imminent. I ushered him, groggy and not quite dressed, to the servants' entrance, apologized, explaining about the maid and that I didn't want to make waves (despite the fact that Spencer had insisted I was free to do "whatever"). I went to the kitchen for a much-needed cup of coffee and introduced myself to Carlotta, who was scrubbing the counter. She snapped her head up toward me and said sharply,

"Mister Forrest told me about you, but didn't say nothin' 'bout no friends. You sure Mister Forrest would like that?"

"Not to worry, Mr. Forrest said I should feel free to use his apartment as I would my own." Not looking too convinced, she went back to her scrub bucket and sponge as if I didn't exist.

After showering off my night of sex, I called Walter, who had said to call when I was ready so he could plan an itinerary of New York night life for the week to come. "Jimmy, mon ami, I caught a glimpse of you on your way out with that Italian sex machine. Your intuition was well-founded. He's rumored to have the biggest salami west of Bologna. Well, dispel the myth for me. Are you or are you not walking bowlegged this morning?"

"To be totally honest with you, I can't remember much. That powder you shoved up my nose really blew me away. I didn't realize what I had done until Spencer's maid woke me up bare naked in bed with this guy."

"Jimmy, relax. Spencer is her meal ticket. Just be glad it wasn't his mother. Oh well, enough of bedtime stories for now. Listen, do you have a tux?"

"Harvey, they don't wear tuxes in Iowa. Bib overalls are about as close as they come. Why?"

"Thursday is the opening of Diana Vreeland at the Metropolitan. Everybody will be there and you will too."

"Who the hell is Diana Vreeland and what is the Metropolitan?"

"Poor baby, you really are green, aren't you, and I love it. Vreeland is only the queen of couture. She puts together an annual fashion show at the Metropolitan Museum of Art. It's a major event. What size are you?"

"Forty regular, why?"

"I'll have Ricci's on 64th have a tux ready for you on Thursday afternoon. Pick it up by six, get dressed and meet me for a drink at eight at the Café Carlyle and we'll head on over."

"But Walter . . ."

"Jimmy, it's all a PR write-off for me, so not another word." I couldn't believe it, my first black-tie event. The only tuxedos I was familiar with were the ones worn at Catholic weddings in Dubuque—beige or robin's egg blue, with ruffled shirts.

Already addicted to the New York night life (and who knew what else), I decided to return to Studio the very next night for a party for Stephen Sprouse. Sprouse was the avant-garde fashion designer on the verge of reviving the Twiggyesque op-art styles of the sixties. Disappointingly, the crowd was strictly downtown: pasty-faced cockney rockers in black cigarette pants, miniskirted, flat-chested, cropped-haired, asexual-looking girls, and a smattering of orange-and purple-mohawked punks — the East Village contingent.

Bored with the freak show, I wandered around aimlessly in fruit-less search for my ideal sexual counterpart. As the crowd thinned, a short, Jewish-looking man staggered towards me with half-closed eyes, working his jaws and licking his lips — obvious signs of too much cocaine and too many quaaludes. He approached with two handsome bartenders and, sans introduction, threw his arms around me as he would a long-lost friend and insisted I return with him and his entourage to his midtown pied-à-terre where the party would continue. "Are your bartender friends also invited?" I said as a joke.

"They're my employees," he slurred, "and the answer is yes." Puzzled, yet intrigued, I followed him through a maze of dingy corridors to Studio's offices where the staff literally bowed to the still-unknown stranger as he proceeded to a big metal desk, un-locked it and took out a supply of pharmacological party favors. I suppose the reason I hadn't recognized him immediately as Steve Rubell, co-owner of the club and King of the Night, was that he hadn't a really remarkable face, and in the photographs I'd seen, its expression wasn't so chemically altered.

With business taken care of, two of his henchmen herded the invited guests out the back door to waiting limousines. I was crammed into one with Halston, his constant companion Bianca Jagger, and D. D. Ryan, an aging socialite with shoe-polish-black hair fixed in a bun with chopsticks. It was beginning to dawn as the two limos pulled up to Rubell's building. As we entered the jar-ringly fluorescent-lit elevator, age lines, eye bags and double chins never visible in the dim of the demimonde sprang starkly to view — the "dueling scars" of years of "battle" in the kingdoms of the night.

At the door, Rubell fumbled with what looked like the complete set of keys for Sing Sing for what seemed like an hour, with no apparent prospect of success. Finally the last of the complex of locks clicked, as we all burst into sarcastic, rowdy applause. We entered into a room that, especially in its lighting, could easily have doubled for Studio's second-floor balcony bar; we were back in the artfully contrived gloom to which we were accustomed, if not addicted. The gargantuan living room was literally a Warhol gallery; mostly portraits whose "originals"—from Mick Jagger to Jackie O.—"hung" (out) at Studio; this gallery was Rubell's personal trophy room.

The dead silence of the room was a bit disconcerting after hours of pounding disco, so Rubell walked as straight as he could over to his stereo and flipped on one of his DJ's choicest mixes. The party was on, Rubell was King, and his courtiers were out in full regalia, ready for a royal debauch. With the "party favors" distributed, everything shifted into truly "high" gear. The haute couture, haute voyeurs, trio of Halston, Bianca and D.D. sat in one corner and watched the *haut*-as-a-kite ensemble shake, rattle and roll.

Suddenly there was a shrill scream from the bedroom hallway. It was Wendy Williams, Texas debutante turned disco dilettante; her friend, spurned by a pro football player, had locked herself in the bathroom and taken an overdose of Seconal. Within minutes police and paramedics were on the scene as guests scrambled to hide their illicit goodies in plants, between couch cushions, and every other place they could think of. I wondered what my parents would do if their son were caught in a highly publicized midtown-Manhattan drug raid. Little did I know then that Rubell made payoffs that made sure the authorities turned a deaf ear and blind eye to his followers' frolics.

Deciding I was once again living too close to the edge, I called it a night—morning, rather—left the party (now resumed after its trivial interruption) and returned to 970 Park, drained yet already eager for my next encounter with the glitterati—Thursday's gala at the Met.

The day arrived, and at four o'clock, I jogged over to the little Italian tailor to try on the tux. Coming out of the changing room, I felt ridiculous, if not desperate. I must not yet be ready for the tuxedo set, I thought: I had the sleek, satin jacket on over a cherished, tattered college athletic shirt and dirty tennis shoes, making me look like a cross between Bert Parks and Moms Mabley. Psyched for the event nonetheless, I left with the tux—but without a thought for whatever accessories it might require—and cabbed it back to Spencer's. After my bath, I combed Spencer's closet for a tuxedo shirt, black tie and black shoes. To my relief (but not surprise), he had plenty of each. I tried on the shirt. The buttons were missing. *All* of them had the buttons missing. Poor Jimmy had never heard of tuxedo studs. I was in a panic. *Where were the goddam buttons?* The best I could come up with were safety pins from Carlotta's sewing box. Then came tying the tie. Improvising brilliantly, I proceeded as with the bow on a Christmas present, then inspected the result. Voilà: Bozo the clown at a funeral. To top (or rather, bottom) it all off, Spencer's innumerable pairs of black shoes were two sizes too small. I ran to the nearest drug store in tux and my brown penny loafers and bought a can of black spray paint. Then I ducked into the nearest alley and sprayed them black. Thus, with spray-painted shoes, safety-pinned shirt and untied tie draping around my neck, I headed for my rendezvous with Walter.

The Café Carlyle was where Bobby Short, the personification of New York class, nightly tickled the ivories to the delight of cafe society. This night, however, due to the gala just blocks away, the show had been canceled and the club was almost deserted. I sat alone at the bar with a five-dollar scotch on the rocks, waiting for Walter but expecting a no-show, moving the drink to and from my mouth carefully to avoid sticking myself with any unfastened safety pins. Walter suddenly burst through the double doors with open arms. "Bonsoir, mon ami Jimmy. What's wrong with your tie? Are you plastered already?"

"Walter, I've never tied one of these before. I must have fumbled for a half hour in front of the mirror. I tried everything from a Cub Scout square knot to shoelace styles. Nothing seems to work."

"Oh, hun. You're not green, you're chartreuse. Here, let me do it for you." We went into the men's room, where within a minute Walter had masterfully worked the tie into *After Dark* perfection.

"Walter, how did you do it?"

"Breeding, my dear Jimmy, breeding. A little artistic genius and a few years of debutante cotillions didn't hurt any, either. And Jimmy, the safety pins? Betsy Johnson would love them, but I doubt they'd make much of an impression on Halston. Where the hell are your studs?''

"Walter, the only studs I know are the ones at the gym." Walter laughed. It was as if I were his Eliza Doolittle and he, my Professor Higgins. He reached out and tweaked my cheek. "Don't worry about it. The lights will be dim and nobody will notice. Just don't get hugsy wugsy with any social matrons. Those bitches are tough as nails and if one pin pops into their boobs, they'll nail you with a lawsuit for assault and battery. Lawsuits are where half their money comes from; that and alimony. Don't let the kissy-kissy lifted smiles fool you; they're a backstabbing, malicious bunch of cunts, just competing with each other with their taffeta and silk originals for a mention in the social columns, gushing over their taste and their bogus philanthropies."

Something told me Walter wasn't crazy about these ladies. Nor had he helped much to calm my nerves, as we climbed into his waiting limousine and headed for the Metropolitan Museum. The immense facade was floodlit, but everything seemed dark compared to the area in front of the entrance. There hundreds of flash bulbs were popping as the invited elite emerged from their limousines. It was like a New York version of the Academy Awards. Now I understood there were two reasons why movie stars wore sunglasses: both for anonymity and to avoid being blinded. I could just imagine my mother sitting under a hair dryer in her beauty shop, opening the *National Enquirer* to a picture of her son emerging from a limousine, in a tuxedo, in Manhattan, and with another man. Her shock would probably blow every fuse in the shop.

As we entered the main reception hall, the glitter overwhelmed me. Giant cornucopias of ice served as centerpieces, surrounded by fresh oysters, caviar, salmon and sundry other delicacies flown in from all over the world to please the most discerning of the international crowd's taste buds. White-jacketed would-be models and actors were racing through the crowd, balancing first-course settings for the sit-down dinner. Everyone milled through the galleries for an hour or so, sipping cocktails, viewing Vreeland's elaborate collection of period costumes, and oozing equally elaborate compliments on each others' gowns and on the exhibit; then dinner was announced.

The seating was carefully marked with placecards, with the inner circle reserved for the richest and most famous, then the lesser notables, and finally the commoners along the outer fringes. Naturally, our table was against the wall next to the busboy station. My company included Walter, two eighteen-year-old Locust Valley lockjawed debutantes, Manfred Beers, a striking Dutch-born model whose face and body graced the pages of every fashion magazine from Albuquerque to Zimbabwe, an obscure embassy dignitary and a couple of titled but fortuneless young Eurotrash men out golddigging for marriage into debutante wealth. The conversation was like a foreign language to me: Everyone had an intimidating air of worldliness. One of the debs, Muffy (yes, some are really called that), chattered away about Junior League cotillions, travel in the south of France, new screenplays, art purchases, etc., etc. My sense of inferiority surfaced with a vengeance. I rather doubted they'd be interested in hearing about keggers in Iowa farm fields, or my meat-cutting experiences at the Pack. So I just sat there on automatic smile, letting their stories go in one ear and out the other, and gazing, enamoured, at Manfred sitting directly across the table.

As mousy Muffy went on and on with a story about falling off Daddy's yacht while sailing off Nantucket, Manfred and I rolled our eyes to indicate to each other our boredom with these twits (and in my case to mask my envy of their charmed lifestyles). The eyerolls were followed by winks and smiles, and suddenly the rest of the evening promised something more than a festival of snobbery and pretense.

After dinner, Peter Duchin and his Orchestra struck up, and portly captains of industry and their arthritic wives hauled their creaking bones onto the dance floor and cranked up their fossilized ballroom dance routines. Muffy grabbed my arm and insisted we join the geriatric set in their slowstep. Catching another wink from Manfred, and afraid of puncturing one of Muffy's already deflated-looking breasts with a safety pin, I respectfully declined and excused myself to go to the restroom. "I'm afraid I've had a bit too much champagne, Muffy, and when nature calls, the bladder must answer."

"Oh, James, you're just too, too." (The adjective itself could be dispensed with, apparently.) "I'll reserve a place on my dance card for when you're feeling a bit more comfortable."

Manfred, who was taking this in, excused himself too and followed me into the men's room.

"Bored?"

"Not anymore."

"Want a toot?"

"Sure, anything to help me deal with that prepped-out douche bag out there."

"Why don't you get rid of her and we'll head over to Studio to do our thing, and then"—giving me another one of his trademark winks—"we'll see what happens."

"Manfred, hold on to your horses, I've got to talk to Walter."

"Oh, is there a thing between you two?"

"No. I'm new to New York; he spotted me on my first night at Studio last week and seemed to think having me around would do things for his PR business, so I'm going along for the ride."

"Well, for an ingenue to the New York scene, you couldn't have chosen better company. Walter's a major PR figure in this town. He makes sure his clients are in the right place at the right time to connect with the right people. We're talking artists with dealers, actresses with studio heads and models with major advertisers and photographers. Most of his money comes from the trust fund set up for him as a baby. This is just playtime for Walter. But his business success doesn't hurt, financially or socially. He's the darling of every socialite in town. To put it crudely, Walter's a great guy, but he's basically a high-class social pimp. We're all buyers and sellers. It only means more business for me from the agencies if the glitterati see me at events like this. The paparazzi love it when they catch a shot of me with Liza or Halston, and it ends up in the tabloids. I've been at this for years now, Jim, so let me give you some advice. Don't become a regular at any place; it dispels the mystique. Be the last to arrive and the first to leave. You don't want to give anyone the impression you're hanging around for the leftovers. With your looks and, judging from the size of your hands and ears, presumably big basket under that tux, you'll be the toast of the town for years to come if you want. Just remember, everything in moderation. This city's got the best of everything—men, money, entertainment, clubs, drugs. But the city can also get the best of you. Walter can show you the social aspects, but I can show you the secret places where the hottest studs in the world dance their tits off all night. You'll feel like a kid in a candy store. No glitter, no social chit-chat, and God forbid, no debs. But for tonight, let's just get out of this mausoleum and make an appearance at Studio in our tuxes, and if I like the way you dance, then I'd like to show you my etchings, so to speak. I can always tell what kind of sex to expect by the moves on the dance floor — and I don't mean the kind of dances you'd do in this joint, with Little Miss Muffy.''

"Sounds tempting, Manfred. You seem to have cultivated the best of both worlds. I have to let Walter know.''

"Jimmy, don't be so obvious. Tell him you had a bad oyster or too much to drink. You don't have to spoil what you can get out of Walter by running off with every sex fantasy and leaving him alone at the mercy of all those drunken society dregs. His whole purpose in bringing you here was to show you off as *his* companion. Can you act? Here, mess up your hair a bit, loosen your tie, pull out one of your shirt tails and look like you've just barfed. Knowing Walter, he'll probably send you home in his limo. I'll be waiting outside and we'll use it to take us to Studio in style. If you stepped out of a cab in a tuxedo at 54, it would be like drinking Dom Perignon with pizza. It ruins the effect.''

I found Walter dragging Muffy around the dance floor to some Tommy Dorsey tune. He danced drunkenly, with the debonaire confidence of Astaire but the skill of a palsy victim. When Muffy and her wallflower friend spotted me they shrieked with schoolgirl giddiness, "Jim, Jim! Come join us! It'll be too, too. We're having a marvey time.''

"Oh, uh, I'd really like to but I'm not feeling too well . . . I'm not used to mixing seafood with alcohol, and I'm afraid it's gotten the best of me. I think I should go home and try to sleep it off.''

Walter grinned his sly one-sided grin, stumbled over and put his arm around me to help me to the door. As I held him up so he could "help me", he said, "Listen, Jimmy, you take some Pepto Bismol, do a little coke and then let Manfred show you the best of the boys in New York. Take the limo and have a ball.''

Reddening in embarrassment at my transparency, I thanked Walter for bringing me to the impressive fete, and confessed my insecurity: "Walter, I have nothing in common with these people. They're rich, famous, and powerful. They might admire my looks but they'd be bored to tears by my conversation. All I can do is sit smiling like a zombie and feeling like a mongrel in a kennel full of purebreds."

"Jimmy, I knew you'd go nuts over Manfred; that's why I made sure you'd be seated at the same table. He is a bon vivant extraordinaire. Besides, his sex is legendary. Now get outta here. Tell the driver to take you wherever, but make sure he's back in an hour to pick me up or carry me out. Don't worry about me, I think you're a hoot. It's like showing Jethro Clampett the Polo Lounge in the Beverly Hills Hotel. Kiss-kiss, ta ta and all that rot. I'll talk to you tomorrow after one to see if Manfred lives up to his reputation. Live it to the hilt, Jimmy!"

Amazed by Walter's hospitality, I bid him adieu and hurried through the great hall to the front steps, where Manfred waited smoking a cigarette and looking as if he had just stepped out of a Dunhill ad.

"Manfred, we got the thumbs up from Walter. It's the third from the left with the TV antennae and 'PR One' vanity plate."

"I know the car very well, Jimmy; it's almost like a second home." We climbed into the back seat, and Manfred pushed a button that raised a smoke glass shield between ourselves and the driver. The bar was amply stocked with Moet. Why not, I thought, with Walter's "Live it to the hilt" still reverberating. What "hilt," or limo ride, was complete without champagne? Totally inexperienced with champagne bottles, I proposed that Manfred do the popping and I the pouring. He went to work, saying, "Champagne is so sexy, don't you think? Opening a bottle to me is like sucking a cock. You have to work at it for a while, slowly, gently, and then when it finally comes, overflowing with foam, you lap up the sweet nectar, savoring every last, intoxicating drop."

I never dreamed I could be given such a hard-on just waiting for a drink. I inched my thigh towards Manfred's, and he reciprocated: a thigh for a thigh. (I love a sense of fair play.) "I can feel something hard down there, Jimmy. I hope you didn't lift some ancient icon from the museum."

"Well, you're half right, Manfred. It's not ancient, but it is lifted, and some people seem to worship it as an icon. And when an art work *this* size is lifted, it's hot. Only a real art-lover — or love-artist — can handle it.''

"Jimmy, an answer like that drives me crazy. Now I don't care if you dance like a hippopotamus; good wit is an even better indicator of good sex. We'll stop at Studio and make one round, just to be seen in our tuxes; then we'll head up to my pied-à-terre on West End Avenue, shed these monkey suits, and have a good, close look at that *object d'art* of yours. I promise you a thorough, professional appraisal.''

The crowd outside Studio seemed twice as large as the first night. Vreeland's opening was highly publicized, and, guessing correctly that the invited would repair to 54 afterwards, half of New York had come to catch a glimpse. Manfred stepped out first, and looking in his tux and slicked back hair like celebrity personified, he strode through the ropes, me in tow, without even slowing down, instantly recognized by Beneke, and apparently also by the gaggle of post-pubescent preppies who stood by squealing with delight. Once inside we made a beeline for the basement, whose gloom was now completely banished by the glow of some of the world's most beautiful models from the Ford, Elite, and Wilhelmina agencies.

Beauty was complemented by art, entertainment and fashion royalty; many of which had arrived just before us from the Met: Halston in black jacket over black turtleneck, Vanderbilt with her permanent smile and trademark hairstyle, Liza Minnelli, Truman Capote, David Hockney, photographers Scavullo and Webber . . . each projecting more than enough *presence* to compete with the mere beauties, whose careers, after all, *they* had made. It was an incestuous bunch, at least as far as careers and reputations went (and no doubt further): While the social shmoozing may have looked like fun and games, the underlying purpose was serious and usually nasty business. Everyone was out for recognition; every word was calculated to advance their own careers — or better still, sabotage someone else's. The saccharine smiles and compliments veiled jealousy and malice. Backstabbing, whoring and ugly gossip went on shamelessly — merely the essential steps in the climb to the top. One whisper into the ear of Scavullo by someone influential that so-and-so didn't have the look, or her hips were too big, or she lacked cheekbones, or was a prima donna to work with, or a major drug addict, or worst of all—"have you seen her cellulite?"— could ruin a budding career. Even supermodel Lauren Hutton would be criticized. The gap in her front teeth was called the result of a jackhammer accident. Her face was lopsided. Her hair was too limp. As though anything *but* these subtle "flaws" distinguished her and singled her out as a star among the cookie-cutter beauties. No matter the profession, having some distinctive trademark was a key to success: With Manfred it was his suave Euro-black-tie-sophisticate look; with Tiegs, her all-American California-surfer-girl look; with Warhol, his catatonic albino look. Oh, and his art . . .

Manfred dragged me through the crowd, introducing me to various notables who gave me little more than a nod and gave all their attention to Manfred, enthralled by his European charm. Cowed by the highbrow crowd's lack of interest in me, I left Manfred and introduced myself to a bejeweled, middle-aged Muffy-type from Greenwich, Connecticut who was trying to guzzle her extra-dry martini as discreetly as possible. " What did you think of the show?" I asked.

"Oh, simply *mar*velous. I wish I had each and every gown to complete my wardrobe. But Justin would just die—he would just *die*. My allowance barely covers my cosmetics, not to mention gowns for events like this. I've worn this dress twice . . . twice!!! Can you imagine? God forbid if anyone notices. By the way, what's your name? You're surprisingly young to be interested in an event like this. Are you a designer?"

"No, ma'am, my name is James Mellon and I was invited to the show by a friend." Well, what's one little letter in a name, if it can make me a member of a great banking family?

"Mellon? Oh my God, are you related to Paul?" (Another of the Pittsburgh Mellons.)

Wanting desperately to be accepted in this crowd, I went on lying through my teeth. "Um, yeah. A distant relative. On my father's side."

"Well, pleasure. I'm Mrs. Endicott."

I would soon have been over my head in BS had Manfred not reappeared and goosed me gently from behind to indicate it was time to go.

Bug-eyed with coke, and with the evening's madness, Manfred and I bailed out of a cab in front of his Upper West Side apartment. The cracked marble floor and chipped rococo mirrors of the lobby testified to a faded grandeur. The burled walnut-paneled elevator inched its way to the top floor at a snail's pace. Inside, Manfred's apartment looked like a male bordello: etchings of male nudes, leopard skin rugs and marble and crystal obelisks filled the dimly lit room, as if each piece was a trophy for some sexual conquest.

"Now we can start the evening. What can I get you to drink?"

"Manfred, I've had enough alcohol to fuel a 747."

"Well, then let's get to it. Come on. Let me show you the room where it all happens. Even sleep, occasionally."

It had an emperor-size bed with a mirrored ceiling. Coke vials, dildos and cockrings, and a library of porn movies filled the shelves above the bed. I knew then I was in the company of one of the world's most famous models *and* Lotharios. And I wanted to discover all the erotic knowledge Manfred had accumulated over the years. I shed my tuxedo and unfastened my safety pins in the bathroom. When I emerged Manfred was naked. Keeping my priorities straight, I looked first at his penis.

I got a shock. It was big. That was fine. That was great. That wasn't the problem. The troubling thing was, it didn't appear to have a head.

What was wrong with it? Was this deformity the result of an accident — a carelessly aimed kitchen knife during a wild session of nude cooking, perhaps — or simply an unfortunate birth defect? I had never seen an uncircumsized penis. The fires of my libido were instantly dampened. Still, my determination to add the otherwise flawless and unquestionably famous Manfred to my list of conquests won out. To make matters worse, a smell, none too pleasant or invigorating, reached my nose from what seemed to be the direction of the same vital yet troubled region of Manfred's anatomy. The man was too stoned to think to wash.

I knew if I betrayed any revulsion, Manfred's offer to show me the hottest of New York's male underworld could be in jeopardy. And any suggestion that he retreat to the bathroom to freshen up would be as insulting as telling Joan Crawford to take acting lessons. So, I attempted to please as best I could without gagging, telling myself that, just as with my drug-induced experience with the Italian the previous night at Spencer's, I wouldn't remember much next morning. In the event, almost before the monster organ had risen, it set again, its "day" cut short by the accelerated clock of coke. All of Manfred's frantic piston strokes and profuse sweating couldn't raise it from the dead. He finally collapsed in exhaustion and frustration. "Goddamn it, I guess champagne mixed with coke is an anti-aphrodisiac. Well, we're not getting anywhere. Let's just take a lude and call it a night. I'm sure I'll be in much better form in the morning."

He reached into his bedside pharmacy and fished out a couple of the pills. When I hesitated, he said if I didn't take one I'd be walking around in circles all night. I decided coke, booze and pot were enough for one night. Besides, I wasn't looking forward to Manfred's vile bratwurst for breakfast next morning. I faked the swallow and waited till he looked good and comatose; then, not wanting to blow my entrée to Manfred's subterranean club world (any more than I wanted to blow Manfred), I left a note on my pillow: "Thanks, Manfred, it was great, but I had to get back to Spencer's to clean the place up before he gets home, or I'll find myself out on the street. I'll take a raincheck for breakfast in bed. Call, stud."

Manfred was right about wandering around in circles all night. Back across town at Spencer's I couldn't sit still, much less lay down and sleep. I walked around the apartment, played the piano, thumbed mindlessly through magazines, wrote illegible, braggadocious letters to friends back at school, and peered into mirrors, admiring myself and simultaneously checking for signs of the wear and tear of unbounded hedonism.

Spencer returned from High Point in midmorning to find me snoring on the couch in the den, still in my tux, while a bright-orange-faced Captain Kangaroo bantered with Mr. Green Jeans on the flickering television.

"Well, dear boy, from the looks of it, you certainly didn't need me to show you the town. How in the queen's name did you end up at a black tie affair your first week?"

"Spencer, this whole weekend has been like a wonderful surreal dream come true. No wonder Eva bitched and moaned about being dragged off to Hooterville." (I wouldn't mention *Green Acres* again, but seeing the TV on reminded me.)

"I presume from that comment, Jimmy, that you've had your first nibble from the smorgasbord?"

"Actually, Spencer, I had a bit of salami and a bit of bratwurst, although the bratwurst left me with indigestion. I think I'd rather stick with good old American hotdogs. Jumbos, at least."

"Better make sure you've got the buns for it. Jimmy, you are too much. Well, you'll probably like my roommate. He's coming back from St. Thomas end of the week and you're right up his alley, and I don't mean bowling. Just a forewarning: Bob's an ex-Harvard football jock, smart as a whip, handsome and horny as a devil, but he can be mean as hell if you cross him. He's squashed many a tight end in his time. But not to worry, Jimmy; I'll make sure he doesn't squash yours—except on request."

That squashed my end of the conversation, as I was still too sleepy for repartee. I thought it wise to inform Spencer of Carlotta's discovery of me and the salami two mornings earlier, before she did. He waved it off. "Oh, don't worry about it. If Carlotta had half a brain, she'd have blackmailed me for half my ownership in Forrest. I just make her Christmas a little greener than most and she don't tell nuthin' to nobody." (Nevertheless, Carlotta's attitude toward me thereafter was similar to the doorman's: I didn't exist.) "Now," Spencer continued, "it's time to show you *my* New York. Forget salami and bratwurst. How about something a bit more refined? Does French suit you?"

"Well, from what I've seen, the women are very elegant. Unfortunately the men seem very similar. So I think I'll pass."

"Jimmy, I meant dinner. I'll bet the closest you've come to French food is french fries and french toast. There's a place in the mid-Fifties called La Caravelle. It's my grandmother's favorite when she comes into town. It's a little stuffy, but the food is indescribable."

"So are my finances. Spencer, I can't afford—."

"Stop, not another word. You are my guest. Meet me here at seven. We'll have a quick drink and head over. Wear coat and tie and be ready."

Doing the best I could with the limited wardrobe I had crammed into my Samsonite, I unfolded a two-sizes-too-small double-knit blue blazer, a remnant of high school graduation; worn and scuffed penny loafers, and a white short-sleeved shirt I'd bought at a Chicago thrift shop for my aborted summer stint at Chez Harvey. This time at least I didn't have to deal with safety pins — only with prickles of embarrassment at my hopelessly middle-American clothes — duds in the true sense. I racked my brain for some way to garnish the outfit with some style. Spencer arrived from work dressed for dinner. The contrast was crushing: in his brass-buttoned Saks blazer, Gucci loafers and Cartier tank watch, Spencer was the personification of New York class. I, on the other hand, was pure scum and yearned to rid the world of my worthless, poorly-dressed carcass. But I hadn't had enough sex yet.

As we entered the restaurant, the maître d' nearly collapsed in servile fawning over Spencer, showering him with compliments, inquiring after the health of his grandmother (probably worried the old crone would check out, depriving him of a long-time patron).

When he'd finished groveling, the maître d' snapped his fingers at a waiter, who brought us an encyclopedic wine list and recited a list of evening's specials longer than and as French as the *Chanson de Roland*. Spencer handled everything as smoothly and casually as if he were ordering at McDonald's. I, of course, was lost, the study of French gastronomy having somehow been omitted from the Chicago Urban Studies program. Brilliant jokes aside, I had no patience for the type of people I'd met there who regarded any luxury or fine living as a form of social injustice. They failed to understand the trickle-down effect of, say, a hundred-dollar dinner expenditure. The waiter who balletically maneuvered the silver trays of food from the kitchen would be downstreaming tips to the busboys who shlepped the dirty dishes back. Part of the bill paid the dishwashers' salaries; another went to the wholesalers. Families would be fed, kids sent to college. In short, the *Cabaret* School of Economics got it (almost) right: money, *circulating*, makes the world go round. Now, if the rich hoarded all their money like Scrooges, then the radicals' critique might be justified. What they needed was a course in Keynesian economics. Instead, "rebels" like my Chicago roommate Ken went on trying to relieve the guilt of their lifelong privileges — European summer camps, sports car graduation gifts, country clubs — by pretending to champion the poor and espousing crackpot theories of liberation.

The waiter brought a bottle of wine that looked like it predated the French Revolution, uncorked it and offered it to Spencer to taste. He went through the whole routine and nodded approval. My own experience with wine consisted of communions at Holy Trinity Lutheran Church in Dubuque, and that only on my parents' insistence. Given the option, I would rather have drunk Pepto Bismol. The wine Spencer had chosen was definitely not for the neophyte. With rather less gusto than Socrates downing his hemlock (a Chateau Thebes 486 B.C., I believe), I forced myself to drink. I too had a point to prove: I wanted to show Spencer that my taste in drink was a bit more sophisticated than beer blasts in Iowa farm fields.

Spencer had been right about this restaurant being stuffy. In two senses. It was a miracle that the geriatric clientele survived their meals without oxygen tents; any tantalizing smells that might have been emanating from the kitchen were drowned by the fumes of pipes, cigars, and sickeningly sweet perfume.

Our waiter lifted the cover of a silver dish to reveal what was called the "appetizer" but what I would have called regurgitated dog food. I poked at the pieces of meat and asked Spencer what it was. "If this is Rocky Mountain Oysters, I'll pass thank you. I had my fill of pig balls working for my father."

"It's escargot, Jimmy."

"What the hell is ess cargo?"

"I'll tell you later. Just trust me and enjoy. It's one of the world's great delicacies. And it's full of protein — good for those muscles of yours."

Always aiming to please, I stabbed one of the slimy bits and placed it in my mouth, hoping for the best. It practically melted in my mouth and slid down my throat. Exquisitely rich, buttery and garlicky, it seemed to signify, no less than the fete at the Met or the basement of 54, how far I'd come from Dubuque. It also contained almost as much wine as my largely untouched glass — as did the main course, Coq au Vin. This was followed by a dessert of rum brulée. Aperitifs before dinner, wine during, booze-soaked dessert and liqueurs after — good thing for the rich that they could afford posh detox clinics.

The bill came and Spencer fumbled for his gold American Express card, adding his usual 25 percent tip to the three-figure total. Just another tax write-off on the Forrest company books.

"Okay, Spencer, dinner's over—what's ess cargo?"

"You liked it, didn't you?"

"Cut the crap, Spencer. Spit it out."

"Well, that's just what I'm afraid you'll do if I tell you."

"I can take it."

"Okay, brace yourself. Snails."

"You mean like the slimy scavengers that cleaned the guppy poop from my fish tank as a child? That's what's now in my stomach?" I was faced with a difficult decision. Did I part company with the offending mollusks right there at our table, onto the table of withered old Mr. and Mrs. Gotrocks adjacent, or did I display true Old World manners and save it until we were at the door bidding the maître d' adieu?

The latter gave an encore performance of kowtowing, accompanied by a Gallic torrent of merci beaucoups and au revoirs, as he opened the door for us, lest Monsieurs Forrest et Melson injure themselves with any undue exertion. A cab had been called and was waiting at the curb. "Now it's your turn," Spencer said as we climbed in. "Why don't you show me a bit of *your* New York? How about taking me to Studio?"

While I couldn't care less what impression I made on the old fossils at La Caravelle, I wasn't about to be seen at Studio looking like I stepped out of a J. C. Penney catalogue. Furthermore, a night at 54 was bound to crank up Spencer's libido. I wanted by all means to get Bud out of my mind through sex with New York's best; but not with Spencer. Living at his place, I didn't want to appear to be his kept boy. I may have stooped pretty low up to this point, but I still stopped short of selling myself. I said, "I think I'll take a raincheck. I'm afraid those snails were all the excitement my stomach and I can handle for one evening."

"I'm sorry, Jimmy. For your gastronomic . . . deflowering, I should have ordered something a bit simpler, like filet mignon."

"You know, Spencer, up until last year I thought filet mignon was fish, and I hate fish, so I never ordered it."

At a loss for words at first, Spencer finally suggested I spend at least one more semester at his "finishing school," which he also referred to as "The Forrest Ward for the Wayward Wicked."

The doorman at 970 Park gave us his usual greeting—a salute for Spencer, the evil eye for me. Upstairs, Spencer insisted on another round of drinks—this time Stingers. Then he dimmed the lights, lit the fire and put on a romantic old Patti Page album. I knew what was next. Drink in hand, he snuggled up to me on the couch and toasted the evening.

One sip and I understood the significance of the drink's name. As for the ingredients, my best guess was rum, turpentine, laundry bleach and insect repellant. At any rate, someone seemed to be holding a blowtorch to my face, occasionally moving it down to my stomach and even my toes.

"Jimmy, did I say something to embarrass you? You're red as a beet."

"Spencer, are you trying to kill me or what? Did you make these drinks at your bar or in Carlotta's cleaning closet? This stuff could unclog drains. I just hope it kills the slimy escargot I still feel crawling around in my stomach. After tonight, I'll be lucky to still have a liver."

There was an awkward silence, during which I felt his eyes fix on me. I fixed mine on the fire and anything else to avoid contact. I sat stiffly, guilt-ridden yet unwilling to give the one thing I had and which he deserved as repayment for his lavish hospitality.

He drained the last of his Draino, put down the Baccarat crystal glass, and making a face like a carp, pressed his lips against mine. He was breathing heavily and practically drooling. I recoiled from his breath—a mixture of the garlicky food, the wine and the Stinger; adding to the bouquet, I could still smell the restaurant's special blend of stale perfume, mothballs and stogies wafting from our clothes. Somehow sensing my lack of enthusiasm—perhaps because I turned away and shuddered—Spencer looked at me and quietly pleaded: "Just once, Jimmy?"

Calculating that if I didn't acquiesce to at least a quick mutual masturbation, I would probably be on the next plane back to Chicago, I unzipped my pants. I wondered what celebrities and studs I had missed that night at 54. I was hopelessly addicted to the New York night life, and would do whatever was necessary—was *at that moment* doing what was necessary — to ensure its continuation. Perhaps I had always had talents for manipulation, exploitation, and deceit; yes or no, New York was serving as Bachelor's program, graduate school, and internship.

When I awoke late the following morning, Spencer was still out cold. First I called Manfred to let him know I was ready for his guided tour of the "underworld"; then I sifted through the dresser for my most cherished Northwestern tank top, sweats and faded blue jeans jacket, and headed out across the park to the West Side "Y" to burn off the previous night's calories. This "Y" was notorious for its postworkout steam baths, where men sat naked, just barely visible in the clouds of steam, moaning, stroking themselves, playing with themselves with one hand and rubbing their sweaty torsos and rippled stomachs with the other, turning themselves on and hoping to attract interested second parties. Seamy as the scene was, it did arouse me. But I used to criticize Mort's sleazy activities at the Julien Hotel in Dubuque, and that sort of thing still repelled me. Besides, steam bath sex was known as a medium for sexually transmitted diseases. So I just watched the lowlifes do their thing. It didn't occur to me that some of these same faceless figures would be among my prime candidates for bedtime partners that very night as they strutted their stuff at the clubs, and that they included Wall Street bankers, lawyers and socially prominent WASPs like Spencer. Even in New York, anonymous acts were the only means of protecting reputations and careers, even if that required stooping to this level. But these were the days when anonymous sex seemed to entail no greater risk than a Herpes blister — a misfortune taken about as seriously as a stubbed toe.

Back at Spencer's, I found messages waiting for me on his answering machine from Walter, the Italian, and Manfred. Walter could be put on hold for future social events. The Italian could offer nothing more than a repeat performance, so his call would not be returned. Manfred, however — my key to the hidden underworld of clubs — I called back immediately. We agreed that he would pick me up that night at 1 a.m. He advised me to nap ahead of time and to set my alarm for midnight to leave time for pushups, situps, curls, and primping. The actual dressing wouldn't take long: "You've seen gay porn, right, Jimmy? Dress down and dirty.

Faded 501s, a beat up old tank. I don't mean to sound dictatorial, but if you show up in Polo pastels, Topsiders and button-down shirt, you won't have a snowball's chance of getting into *this* hot spot. It's not a place for pretty young WASPs from Connecticut or the Hamptons. Just think hard, muscular and masculine and you'll be a shoo-in. We're talking serious hedonism and narcissism. I'm sure you won't disappoint.''

The club, Flamingo, surpassed all of Studio's flash, cash and glitz. Hundreds of thousands of dollars worth of state-of-the-art sound and lighting equipment were hidden behind its inconspicuous, dimly lit entrance. Entrée was even more selective than at Studio: none but the most outstanding male specimens that walked the face of the earth stood a chance. Juice and soda were all that was available, but that proved sufficient fuel — along, of course, with massive quantities of drugs — to keep the superbly muscled patrons bumping and grinding into wild frenzies.

I was, however, taken aback by the club's forbidding-looking neighborhood. As we got out of the car, I said, ''Manfred, are you sure you've got the right address? Looks pretty scary to me.''

''That's the point, Jimmy. This place is a secret. If it had the PR and hoopla of Studio, you'd have every wimpy queen from Queens trying to push his way in to rub elbows, not to mention crotches, with the amazing mounds of flesh you're about to meet.

The bouncer looked like a Neanderthal. Standing with massive arms folded, he made Beneke look like Shirley Temple. One swoop of his giant hand could have put a rhinoceros into a coma.

''Nothing to be afraid of, Jimmy. He's harmless as a fly to those who belong; but, beware, those who don't. They call him Slug. Strange, all that brawn and no brains. The only things I've ever heard come from his mouth are 'fuck you, mother fucker' and 'eat shit and die.' Not one of the world's great conversationalists. What would Muffy make of him? She'd probably say, 'Slug, you're just too, too.' Can you imagine him as her dinner companion at the Metropolitan? They'd have to carry her out on a stretcher.''

Thankfully, we breezed past the stoney-faced axeman, and into a dingy lobby that could easily have been mistaken for the basement of Studio. But up two flights of treacherous metal stairs, I thought I had died and gone to homo heaven. Half-naked, gleaming, sweaty gods writhed, humped and bumped in cadence to Don Henley's "Dirty Laundry." Among them could be found every man's physical/sexual ideal. It was a veritable Olympics of narcissism, in which competition (and no doubt more) was stiff, the gold going to those who drew the most attention with their "come fuck me" looks. Most were in search of that impossible dream, their identical twin. This resulted in clusters of near-clones, their steroidal muscles inflated like Macy's parade floats and flexed for maximum effect (all perhaps in compensation for underdevelopment of the one muscle that *really* counts; pumping iron is no help there!). Marlboro and Budweiser models exchanged compliments on their chiselled facial features and trashed those who lacked them; Columbia and NYU rugby, crew, and lacrosse champions replayed past victories over other Ivy teams, and over sorority girls they had spurned. Sex talk was rampant, the central question being whether one took it "doggie style" or just sixty-nined. The 501 jeans were sandpapered at the crotch to create a "big basket" effect. Finally, as though everyone wasn't horny enough, a menu of drugs was available to boost their libidos another hundred or so horsepower.

Manfred, noticing me salivating and my eyes about to pop out of my head, reached into his wallet and fished out a dried piece of mushroom.

"A bit intimidating for you, James? Here, swallow this and your insecurity will vanish. You'll be floating around in love with everyone as they with you."

"Manfred, the only mushrooms I've ever eaten came out of a can or were sprinkled on pizza. How do you know those strange things didn't grow out of a dung heap somewhere? Look, Manfred, I may be adventurous, but I figure if I play my cards right, I've still got forty or so years ahead. Longevity runs in my family and I'd rather not break the streak. I can just see my mother getting a long distance call that her pride and joy has died in a homosexual New York discotheque from eating a magic mushroom. I think I'll pass."

"Jimmy, look at me. Do I look like a corpse? I've been doing them for years. Trust me. If you don't, you'll just be sitting on the bleachers like a wallflower at a high school homecoming dance. You won't be mentally in sync with the rest of the crowd."

Just as with Walter's coke, I smelled the thing, hoping for some sort of reassurance. At least it was dried and dead; I didn't have to worry about it crawling around in my stomach like the escargot at La Caravelle. What harm could something so innocent and pathetic-looking do? Trusting Manfred, I thrust it into my mouth and quickly washed it down with juice.

Manfred and I walked around the edge of the dance floor, perusing the men as they revved up their jet-fueled engines, pumping to the music. Within minutes, it was as if my every nerve ending was on the verge of ejaculation. My mouth went dry and I excused myself from Manfred to empty my bladder, and, of course, check myself in the mirror. As full as my bladder felt, nothing happened. It was as if the mushroom was literally blocking the way. Only by exerting enough pressure to cause a hernia did a few drops trickle out. I left the stall, looked in the mirror, and stared in shock at a monster with coal-black eyes.

"My eyes! Good God, my eyes! These fucking mushrooms have made my beautiful blue eyes turn black!"

"So what'sa matta wid black eyes? I got 'em and dey don't stop heads from turnin." The eloquent hulk was flexing his pectorals at the next mirror. "What'sa matta man, never done 'shrooms? Don't fuckin' worry 'bout it. By noon tomarra', they'll be back to baby blue. Besides, people won't be lookin' at your eyes, it's strictly muscles and baskets in this joint. Get over it. C'mon, stud, let's go out and strut it. Mickey and Sally are waitin' at the bar and Sally's got the rag. That'll really rev you up."

Mesmerized by the pulsating pecs, my terror about my eyes quickly dissipated. I followed him out to the dance floor where we joined a similar-looking hulkster distinguished by a tatoo around his bicep of a rope tied in a sailor's knot, which when he flexed, became untied. Hanging onto his forearm, the top of her head barely reaching his cockring-pierced nipple, was a woman at least seventy-five in a spandex suit and rhinestone boots: It was Disco Sally again — the legendary diva of the dance clubs. She seemed to know her way around the scene as well as Manfred and Walter combined. How many seventy-five-year-old former Kansas librarian spinsters spent their retirement in New York discos riding the shoulders of massive musclemen and screaming "Whoopie" and "ride 'em cowboy" after inhaling an ethyl-chloride-soaked athletic sock? Not more than a few hundred, I'd bet. As a late bloomer myself (though not *this* late), I empathized with her attempt to make up for a lifetime of emptiness and disappointment with a December spree of self-abandon; if the remaining years were few, at least they would be full.

Mickey and I helped Sally onto her "mount" as the DJ cranked up Gloria Gaynor's "I Will Survive" — Sally's request. With one whiff of her rag, her arms began flailing wildly and she became Clara Bow and Jean Harlow and every other Silver Screen siren she had idolized in her childhood combined. The crowd circled around her, cheering. She seemed destined to go to her grave with an ethyl chloride rag in her mouth and a smile on her face.

I hadn't expected that to occur *immediately*, however; but, thanks to my innocent, pathetic mushroom, Sally now underwent a horrifyingly morbid transformation. First, with her wrinkles and her shrieks, she began to resemble my grandmother watching a Minnesota Vikings game. That was bad enough. Then her flesh began to decay more and more every second. Then everyone else began to decay. The Valhalla of handsome gods became a hellhole of melting monstrosities — then one great many-headed monster threatening to engulf me in an avalanche of putrefying flesh. Sweat poured from my brow. I had to escape. Where was the exit? Where was Manfred? Oh, my god — was I decaying too? Where's the bathroom? Get me a mirror! Panic stricken, I walked or ran to the DJ booth, and asked — or screamed — "How do I get out of here? Where's the door?" The DJ had obviously seen as many "crises" like mine as he'd seen rotations of his turntable.

"Relax, everything will be okay. You're having a bad trip. Something set you off. Just wait. In a few minutes you'll be back on the floor drooling over some stud. Here, take this "lude," it'll cool you down."

One more drug didn't scare me. The way I already felt, given a gun I probably would have pulled the trigger. I gulped it down and stood against the wall with eyes closed, and in no rush to open them.

Don Henley's "Dirty Laundry" began to play again. I felt a wave wash over me, and wash away my nightmare — a huge wave of *pure sex*. I opened my eyes: rotting carrion was firm, inviting flesh again; the monsters were reincarnated back into Adonises. I floated out on the floor and began to dance like a Vegas stripper, caressing my body, thrusting my pelvis Elvis-style like I was in the middle of a deep fuck — feeling as if every eye in the house were on me.

The remainder of the evening was a euphoric blur. My most distinct memory is exiting into the shock of blinding daylight, painfully intensified by my dilated pupils. The cab ride home was Rude Awakening, Phase II. Fully hip to the addled condition of people leaving this club, cab drivers lined up around the block looking to take the passengers for a ride, literally and figuratively; especially if the destination was a Park Avenue address. And I was addled, to say the least, after the "lude." My senses of time and distance were missing in action. I do remember that the driver resembled the meat-cutting redneck in Dubuque who had dumped pig entrails on my head — an interesting coincidence, since this one was to dump on me too: when he finally stopped at 970 Park, he barked, "Twenty bucks, Mack." The bastard must have circled Central Park three times to have run it up so high. But I thought it best not to dispute the issue, for fear of him flooring the pedal to dump me in Harlem or the East River.

Raunchy and foul in torn jeans, sweat and baby oil, I pushed the elevator button and watched the brass pointer count down from the penthouse. The elevator door opened and out came a well-heeled, WASPy, wholesomely smiling couple, much like Thurston and Lovey Howell from *Gilligan's Island*. "Lovey" was obviously taken aback at my appearance and grabbed her husband's arm a little tighter. I offered a sheepish "Good Morning"; "Thurston" answered with a "harumph," knitted brows, and a "Who is this guy?" look at the doorman. The temptation to introduce myself and to describe my night and my preceding few days in complete detail was powerful indeed.

I crawled into Spencer's apartment to find him sipping his morning coffee and reading the Sunday *Times*.

"Jimmy, I see you've discovered Flamingo."

"How can you tell?"

"Please, I'm not blind. You're drenched in baby oil and your pupils are as big as bowling balls, and there's only one place in town that's open all night and through the next morning to get as down and dirty as you look. I think you better take a rest from this before that blond mop of yours turns gray. I'm headed to the Cape tomorrow to visit my family for the Fourth; maybe you'd like to come along. Consider it a detox center."

"Detox from what, Spencer, the escargot?"

He ignored that. "You should be getting over your Chicago friend by now. This might help. Do you think you can shift your libido into neutral for a long weekend of R and R at the beach?"

He didn't have to twist my arm. The mere thought of Spencer's Cape Cod house was as impressive to me as the modest Cape Cod-style bungalow in which I'd grown up was to the factory workers living in the surrounding Levittown-like houses, to whom a few shutters, a cedar shake roof, a chimney, a fireplace, and an Ethan Allen reproduction dining room set were tantamount to descent from the *Mayflower* (and whose own symbols of antiquity were some rusty farm implements, slot machines and Kewpie dolls). Ironic how, in relative terms, my move "up" to New York was a move down in the world.

We crossed the Triborough Bridge at dawn to beat the rush hour. The interstate took us whizzing along the coast, past Greenwich, Mystic and Newport — names that echoed from my high school American history, evoking great oil and railroad fortunes whose present-day heirs I pictured luxuriating beneath the slate roofs and great chimneys I could see towering above manicured hedges, scotch pines and stone walls. Passing signs to the Vanderbilt mansion in Newport, I was pinching myself in an unsuccessful effort to stifle my whining pleas for a quick detour.

"Jimmy, I'd love to but we really should get there before the fog rolls in. The road to Hyannisport can be a bitch in ten-foot visibility, and at this time of year that's nightly."

I sat pouting and soon nodded off to sleep. I awoke at the toll bridge entering the Cape. Spencer was right about the fog: it was thick as mud. I imagined lurking within it the ghosts of all the witches and homosexuals burned at the stake around here in the seventeenth century. Spencer was whipping around hairpin turns in fifth gear, eager to get home and tired of having had to do all the driving himself (my Iowa license was zapped at St. Olaf because of a mountain of unpaid parking tickets). Night had fallen when, after endless twists and turns, we pulled into an unremarkable-looking driveway.

"Spencer, there's a 'Do Not Enter' sign there. Are you sure about your directions?"

"Don't worry about it, its always there."

I thought nothing further of it for the moment. We parked and got our luggage out of the trunk. The house itself was a mere twenty feet from the driveway, behind a knee-high white picket fence. Through the fog, all I could see of the house was a modest-looking green-shuttered door, much like the entrance to our house in Dubuque but without the latticed, ivy-covered porch. I felt a bit like the dupe of some fly-by-night tour operator. Surely Spencer had taken a wrong turn in the fog — or was playing a tiny joke; we would pay a brief visit to some poor relation, then back up and return to one of the sumptuous palaces we'd passed en route.

We entered a miniscule foyer. "Well, here we are," Spencer chirped. "What do you think?"

"Well . . . I . . ."

"Spencer, is that you?" Mrs. Forrest breezed gracefully into the adjacent reception room dressed in a loud but elegant Lily Pulitzer floral print that owed a debt to Monet. She grasped Spencer's shoulders and raised her cheek an inch or two toward his — hardly a kiss; more a well-practiced gesture. *Her* entrance, at least — unlike the house's — began to meet my expectations of elegance and restore my shaken faith. Then she offered me a limp hand and a forced smile that seemed to mask a "Who in God's name are you?" as though instincts told her, even before I spoke, that I was not of the Forrest ilk; as if she detected the odors of Iowa pig manure *and* my night at Flamingo. But Spencer had thought of everything. Without skipping a beat, he introduced me — to his mother as well as to myself: "Mother, meet Jim Melson. He just flew in from Chicago yesterday for an on-campus interview at Columbia and thought he'd catch a ride up with me to visit his brother Skip in Boston who prepped with me at Choate."

Well. I seemed to be moving up in the world after all.

Chapter 6

Moving Up in the World: Cape Cod

Wealth is not without its advantages.

—John Kenneth Galbraith

Satisfied with my credentials, Mrs. Forrest's suspicious gaze gave way to a too-toothy, classically New England smile. While it was well known that many a WASP, weary of the cocktail set at the Hyannisport Club and horny from the summer sun, would end up at the "P-town" (Provincetown) bars, presenting a gay lovemate to the family was unheard of, especially on a holiday weekend when staunch traditions prevailed.

"Well, James, glad to have you. We're very informal here, so make yourself at home. What would you like to drink?" Into an intercom, she said, "Bertha, come take drink orders." Within seconds, a massive black woman in uniform and support hose shuffled from the kitchen. Bertha made Carlotta look petite. How they provided a uniform for her was beyond me; they must have dyed a circus tent white. Perhaps her figure resulted from functioning as the family's leftover food depository.

"Well, look at you, Mister Forrest, doncha' look mighty fine," she beamed, engulfing Spencer in an eye-popping Southern Baptist bearhug. Bertha had been with the family since Spencer's birth and had nursed him through his childhood while his mother was attending social functions and choosing fabrics for the Forrest lines. To the Forrests, Carlotta and Bertha were members of the family, very much à la television's "Hazel." Whereas, to my former Urban

Studies colleagues, I reflected, the employment of *any* servants amounted to feudalism, and *black* servants, to slavery.

We made our way into a sizeable living room where Spencer's father was dozing in a wingback chair in front of a walk-in-sized fireplace hung with antique bed warmers, trivets and cauldrons, his reading specs askew and a *New England Journal* resting on his portly bourgeois belly. Mrs. Forrest leaned forward. "Miles, wake up, Spencer is here." Miles awoke with a porcine snort, his eyes bloodshot and bagged, the rewards, I supposed, for typical WASP alcoholic overindulgence.

"Wha . . . , Wha . . . , Spencer my boy, we'd just about given up on you."

"Miles, this is James Melson," said Mrs. Forrest. "He's just interviewed at Columbia, he's a brother of one of Spencer's old Choate alums and he's on his way up to Boston to visit him."

"Ah, pleasure, good man, good man. Any relative of Choate stock is top drawer. Welcome to our humble abode."

His style might have been a near-parody of a 1930s drawing-room comedy, but the "humble abode" part was true. A quick tour before bedtime took us down long hallways floored in worn wide-plank pine, past numerous but modest bedrooms furnished in Early Thrift Shop. Faded chintz drapery, creaking floors and peeling paint prevailed throughout, the work of centuries of unheated dry winters and humid summers. A slant-roofed suite with fireplace, kelly green carpeting, and plain, fraternity house atmosphere, I was told, was the master bedroom. Visiting family members already occupied the other eight bedrooms, so I was to stay in a room on the far side of an institutional-sized kitchen. Once servants quarters, the room was done up in jail-cell minimal with bunk beds, dresser, pitcher and bowl. As Spencer brushed cobwebs filled with dead bug carcasses from the ceiling, a wave of pungent mildew odor made me gag.

"Spencer, this place could have been the set for the attic in Hitchcock's *Psycho*. How can your family run a prestigious furniture company and then fill their rooms with furniture from a motel liquidation sale?"

"Well, Jimmy, my parents are getting older and it's rare that we have an overflow from the main house bedrooms. My parents probably haven't even seen these rooms in two years. Open the window; let the breeze caress your bare body. The salty air will cleanse all the poisons you've managed to consume these last few weeks. You dealt with the mushrooms pretty well; a little mold and mildew isn't going to hurt any.''

"*Mold and mildew?* There are probably *mushrooms* growing in here!''

"Well, if you find any, save them,'' Spencer laughed. "I'm waking you up at the crack of dawn for the royal tour. Now I'm off to my quarters. Good night.''

I assumed the "royal tour" meant backtracking to the mansions we had passed on the freeway. It couldn't be anything around here — not if the neighboring houses resembled John Irving's *Hotel New Hampshire* as much as this one did. Where were the marble floors, the old master paintings, the Persian rugs? I was also baffled by Spencer's comment about his "quarters" — and that he seemed to be heading out the back door.

"Spencer, aren't you going the wrong way?''

"No, my place is over the garages. It's the chauffeur's quarters when my grandmother is here alone. It's my only means of maintaining my privacy, not to mention my sanity, when my family is underfoot. You've heard the creaky floors. The sound reverberates throughout the whole house and any attempt at sneaking in or out would scare the bejesus out of my mother. She sleeps light as a feather ever since we had a series of burglaries at our house in Wellington. She keeps upgrading the alarm system; I swear the next step will be a crocodile-filled moat. With one creak she'd flip the switch next to her bed and this place would be crawling with cops. With a place over the garage I can bring people home and not risk jolting my mother out of bed with her billy club and mace while I'm in the middle of screwing around. Besides, we have some fairly well-known neighbors whose reputations we try to keep untarnished. Photographers and media vultures are lurking around the house night and day just to catch a shot of some scandalous act for the tabloids. My mother would have a stroke if she turned to page six of the *Post* and saw a picture of some terrified bare-assed trick with a hard-on running out of our front door, not to mention overhearing dinnertime scuttlebutt at the Hyannisport Club about strange bedfellows coming and going at all hours over at the For-rests'. You know, Jimmy, the main part of this house is the oldest structure in Hyannisport, and it's been said that a church deacon was caught performing fellatio on the original owner's twelve-year-old son and was subsequently hung in the town square. While times may have changed, my neck may not be hung but it certainly would be wrung. Talk about rednecks in Dubuque — well, where do you think their ancestors came from? Here you wouldn't find farm ani-mal carcasses hanging from meat hooks, but tarred and feathered homosexuals. The Cape prides itself on its staunch traditions that have remained intact for centuries, and they include remnants of Mayflower morality. But don't worry, Jimmy, the death penalty for sex acts went out with the Revolution, and witch burning.''

Spencer left me unable to sleep, his gruesome little historical anecdote echoing in my ears. According to ghost stories, it was often those who'd met with violent deaths whose spirits hung around causing trouble. Would old Deacon Pederast, horny as hell after two or three hundred years of disembodiment, sense my pres-ence and, so to speak, reveal himself to me? Manfred's pungent pubes would seem positively pristine compared to someone who hadn't washed in three centuries. I lay on the musty bed with a mothball-reeking blanket over my head, listening to the creak of the old structure — or was it the floorboards? The ocean breeze picked up, and through the window there suddenly blew a whisp of fog. Goose bumps crawled up my arms and legs, and I felt the hairs there (and nothing else) stand erect, as though someone — or thing — were passing a static-charged hand lightly over my flesh. The deacon was back for his revenge! He would tie his noose to my manhood and force me to leap out the open window to a gruesome combination death/castration! I finally got the courage to jump out of the bed, armed with the pitcher, to switch on the light. Jimmy, get a grip, there are no such things as ghosts. Old houses make noises when they settle, just like your father when he settles on his couch in the den to listen to Pavarotti. Nevertheless, for the rest of the night the light stayed on and the door bolted.

The early morning sun had burned off the fog, and through the paned-glass window I looked out onto a vibrant symphony in green, blue and white. Motor yachts and sailboats were already out for their glorious Fourth cruises. I skipped down the steep, winding back stairs and out the servants' entrance, where, at the sight of four rambling white framed houses shuttered in green and roofed in cedar, I experienced a déjà vu of at least seven on the Richter scale — or whatever the scale is. Everything looked so incredibly familiar. But how could I have seen this place before? Was I a reincarnation of the deacon's young victim? I'd received communion from clergymen in my time, but not *that* kind. A bored-looking uniformed security guard sat in an unmarked blue Chevy in the drive, paging through the *Boston Globe*. Noticing me out of the corner of his eye, he jumped out and barked, with hand on holster, "What are you doing here? This is private property. No one's allowed behind the barrier."

Boy, Spencer wasn't exaggerating about his mother's security paranoia. The Chicago Art Institute or the Metropolitan, maybe; but why would this simple, cheaply furnished house need an armed guard?

"I'm a guest at the Forrests', sir."

"Okay, you're clear."

I went back in through the servants' entrance and met Spencer coming into the kitchen for his morning caffeine fix.

"I just met your security guard. I passed inspection, but his gun and billy club were just a bit intimidating. Spencer, I know you're going to think this is off the wall, but I think I've seen this place before. Why do these houses look so familiar?"

"I don't know. Do you have any Kennedy blood in you?"

"What do you mean?"

"The house across the street is Ethel's, next to Ethel's is Rose's and behind Rose's is Jackie O.'s. Ours was Jean Kennedy and Steven Smith's before my parents bought it. Don't be obvious, but if you look behind you, you'll see Rose being wheeled up the drive for her morning air."

I turned to see a shriveled and blanketed old woman, well into her eighties, sitting in a wheelchair being pushed by a white uniformed nurse. The matriarch of the famous first family flashed an unmistakable Kennedy smile.

"Good God, Spencer, you mean. . . ." A white BMW came whizzing by the barricade, blaring its horn at Rose and screeching into Ethel's driveway. Members of Ethel's clan came bounding out in white tennis togs, pushing, shoving and swearing. Between the white house, white car and white clothes, the scene looked like a commercial for Clorox bleach. No thesaurus could express how dumbfounded, awestruck, astounded, astonished, amazed, startled, stunned, stupefied and staggered I was at my unexpected proximity to America's royal family.

"Spencer, why didn't you tell me?"

"Because I didn't invite you here to gawk at the Kennedys. I asked you up to enjoy the Fourth of July with me and my family. If word got out in New York that I had unrestricted access to my family's beach house in the Kennedy compound, there'd be a line of fags for blocks in front of 970 Park every weekend hoping to tag along for a good look at John John and I'd sit here solo on the beach, used and abused. I saw that smile on your face when I mentioned John John, Jimmy. Don't get any ideas about bedding him down. You get within a hundred feet of him and you'll have secret service men all over you."

"Well, that might prove more interesting than John John."

"Behave and go put on your most outrageous pastels, we're invited to Harc and Lloyd's, a.k.a. Hansel and Gretel, for brunch. You'll get a true taste of old-guard WASP fags. They're a hoot and a half. They live over in Osterville on the bay side. Money over there goes back as far as Midas himself."

Spencer and I drove through a quaint shopping area dotted with antique stores, Lili Pulitzer outlets and French pastry shops until the rotary spun us onto the Osterville route. Within minutes, massive colonial and Tudor houses appeared, each of hotel-like proportions and protected behind gated and guardhoused walls. We passed a stone marker that Spencer said indicated the outer border of Harcourt Carver Meadows III's property, through which we continued to drive for what seemed like miles. We passed a vacant and dilapidated sprawling white structure on our left.

"Is that it, Spencer?"

"It's theirs, but they don't live there. A little impractical for two, don't you think? Harc's grandfather built that white elephant in the days of the railroad barons. Harc and Lloyd live in a modest three bedroom that used to be the caretaker's house. It's just up the road." As Spencer pulled into the circular driveway, tooting the horn of his canary yellow VW "Thing," a late-fifties-ish couple garbed in patriotic red, white and blue emerged from the house, each with a sparkler in one hand and a Bloody Mary in the other, swishing and swaying with the hypercampiness of a Benny Hill queer routine. In the great we-get-plastered-at-the-drop-of-a-hat WASP tradition, the two had obviously gotten a sizeable head start on us; indeed, their blue-veined noses and bloodshot eyes almost made the bunting colors they wore redundant. Determined to outdo Pearl Mesta at playing the hosts in their antique-filled love nest, immediately upon entrance Harc dipped a garish sterling silver ladle into a toilet-bowl-sized crystal punch bowl filled with Bloody Mary mix of explosive strength, while Lloyd, in a red-and-white-striped apron, brought out finger sandwiches, canapés and puff pastries arranged as painstakingly and delicately as a house of cards.

"We hope you don't mind the lightness of the meal, but Harc's on a diet," Lloyd chortled as the embarrassed Harc pulled his size-forty yachting pants up over his paunch, almost to his chest.

Not about to let Lloyd get away unanswered, Harc retorted, "You'll have to excuse the strength of the Bloodys, Jimmy, but Lloyd has an extreme distaste for liver and he's doing his best to get rid of his." And so the catty insults kept volleying back and forth like a Ping-Pong ball.

"So, Jimmy, you're really one of those legendary corn-and-cattle-fed boys we've always fantasized about but were never fortunate enough to come across," Harc said, eyeing me head to toe. "Which side of the Mississippi is Dubuque on anyway?" he added, feigning naiveté.

"North, of course." (Guffaws.)

"Very quick-witted, Jimmy. I'm sure you'll do quite well in New York."

"I think you've got that slightly mixed up, Harc," Spencer interjected. "Don't you mean, I'm sure he'll *do New York* quite well? That's more appropriate. You can take it from me." He paused. "Although *he* won't, unfortunately."

I flushed at this advertisement of my sexual rapacity. At the rate word was spreading up the Eastern Seaboard, I'd soon be a legend in Labrador. Noticing my unease, a now-soused Lloyd warbled,

"Nothing to worry about, Jimmy, you're a healthy young man with a healthy young libido. Just keep it clean and stay away from those ethnics and exotics. God knows what kind of microbes they carry around. Stick to clean-cut all-American boys like Harc and myself. Whoops! Freudian slip."

"Forgiven, Lloyd." (But not for the typical misuse of 'Freudian slip,' I added silently.) "The red, white and blue just went to your head." Especially the Bloody red.

Judging from how much Harc, and especially Lloyd, had eaten — and drunk — they seemed to regard the Fourth of July as a mid-summer Thanksgiving. All that was left of the heaping plates of finger foods were a few flaky crumbs of puff pastry, which Harc was making short work of with his fingertips. His pants had now slipped back well below the belt line. Lloyd whipped the plate from under his fingers. "Why don't you lick the goddamn plate so I don't have to do the dishes? You just don't know when to quit, do you?" Then he stormed out towards the kitchen, emitting sarcastic piglike snorts.

Harc sat blank-faced and teary-eyed, as stung by the truth of Lloyd's taunts as by their unkindness. "You'll have to excuse Lloyd. It just goes to show what happens after twenty years of too much booze, too many wrinkles and not enough compassion." The poor man buried his face in his hands and broke into gasping sobs. The pitiful sight awakened painful memories: in the snubbed and wounded fatso, I saw myself in my youth. Disturbed, I excused myself and went to the bathroom, leaving Spencer to give solace. The bathroom walls were covered with photos of Harc and Lloyd at various points in their lives — smiling and with arms around each other in their younger years, gradually giving way to stiff, unsmiling arms-folded, almost Victorian poses in the later pictures; hard, sobering evidence of how a relationship, no less than its partners, developed wrinkles, a paunch, and heart trouble.

When I came back, Spencer stood up and said we had to be leaving for the beach. We both realized that the afternoon would be unsalvageable after the infantile flareup. Spencer too was solemn on the way back to Hyannisport. I said, "Spencer, is this how it becomes?"

"How what becomes?"

"What we just witnessed, ridiculing each other in front of guests, and in my case a total stranger."

"Jimmy, Harc and Lloyd's relationship is well-founded. Granted, the passion may dry up, but they've had over twenty years of happy times together, and they still have each other to treasure the memories with. An occasional alcohol-induced slip of the tongue will be forgotten in an hour or two and it will be back to business and campiness as usual by tomorrow morning. They'd be lost without each other's companionship in their golden years. Let's face it, none of us is ever going to have children or grandchildren to be doting on us. Bickering is probably a lot better than loneliness."

I wasn't convinced. I'd never seen my parents hold hands, much less give each other a passionate kiss. Now Harc and Lloyd's cruel jabs at each other made me wonder more than ever whether years of passion, devotion and giving to one person were worth it, if this was what it came to. Even worse was witnessing the physical decline. I was suddenly glad about my short-term relationships with Scott and Bud. Who wanted to watch, embittered, as they succumbed to sagging paunches, arthritic joints and wrinkled skin? *My* memories would remain frozen in time; retain their Dorian Gray perfection. An aging lover is, after all, an ever-present mirror of one's own mortality.

As Spencer maneuvered the curves to Wianno beach, the salty sea breeze blowing through my hair and caressing my face swept Harc and Lloyd from my mind and filled it with 1960s beach-boy fantasies. The ocean at long last! Waves crashing on endless stretches of fine white sand! Why, it was almost enough to make me stop missing the mighty Mississippi oozing past Dubuque's bluffs, rich with mud and ripe with raw waste dumped by the Pack. Bronzed, taut bodies bobbed in the surf, waiting for the perfect wave to hang ten on their boards; others tackled each other on the sand in pursuit of a well-worn football. A totally different male style prevailed on the Cape beach than among the trash that littered the Oak Street beach in Chicago. Here were no vulgar, blatantly bulging monokinis. Crotches and buttocks were conservatively covered in baggy Brooks Brothers bermudas and Ivy gym shorts, leaving the fantasy to the eye of the beholder. I felt naked in my navy-and-gold-striped Speedo, and I dashed into the surf for cover. I attempted a few strokes of "fly" to impress Spencer and the oblivious jocks, but a near-tidal wave carried me back onto the beach and deposited me katywampus at Spencer's feet, and as it retracted, it pulled my swimsuit down to my knees. Shell fragments and sand clogged my every orifice. It was as if the ocean had tasted the foul Mississippi on me and spit me out in disgust.

I wasn't going to let a little ocean like the Atlantic humiliate *me*. It was confusing itself with the Pacific. I was full of—well, yes, sand, but also the Hemingway spirit. I knitted my brow, (literally) gritted my teeth, pulled my suit back up ("girding my loins" as they say) and resolved that the ocean must not win. Realizing now that the four-foot breakers were not ideal for swimming laps, and noticing others using their bodies as human surf boards, I attempted to follow suit.

When I washed up with my swimsuit down *this* time, it was at the feet of a gaggle of streaky-haired girls with Ultrabright teeth sitting on their beach towels and tittering at the uncoordinated klutz with the cold-shrunken manhood who couldn't master the waves. I felt like a stripper on 42nd Street whose G-string had broken. The hell with Hemingway. I no longer saw the importance of being Ernest. I just earnestly wanted out. I waded my way back to Spencer, who sat on his towel laughing hysterically.

"Come on, Spencer. Let's get out of here before these prepettes lynch us."

"The last time there was a lynching up here was the deacon, but after a couple hundred years they may well be itching for another. Well, we've got to get back anyway and clean up our act before cocktails with the family. They've invited us to accompany them for the traditional Yale Whiffenpoofer's Fourth of July sunset concert at the beach club and dinner afterwards at the Hyannisport Club."

"Now let's see—is a Whiffenpoofer something to do with woofers and tweeters, or gay dog owners, or some exotic sex act—or all three? I'm game."

"That's right, my parents are going to watch gay dog owners **perform exotic sex acts. Jimmy, it's a men's glee club. And 'glee'** doesn't mean what you probably think, either. Just try to remember one thing: The beach club is not Flamingo. There is no DJ booth.

Mushrooms are not available, nor will you bump and grind. And the Hyannisport Club is the bastion of old guard WASPdom; if you don't have a family crest on your blue blazer, eyebrows will ascend."

"Will John John be there?"

"Jimmy, the Kennedys hardly fit into the WASP category. People around here refer to Kennedys as WICS."

"'Wicks'?"

"White Irish Catholic Scum. They don't have a good name up here."

"That makes three places where the family of our thirty-fifth president has a bad name: Cuba, the Kremlin, and the Hyannisport Club in Cape Cod."

"It's not me, Jimmy—it's the culture up here. They're harder to crack than a granite oyster. First of all, the Kennedys think they own the Cape. Secondly, they are, as you may know, Democrats; everyone else around here is Republican. Thirdly, Chappaquiddick, Marilyn Monroe, Aspen drug overdoses . . . Need I say more?"

Looking *down* on the Kennedys! I was impressed. This was a whole new level of snobbery. I could just imagine the Kennedys moving into Catholic Dubuque's beach enclave (if they *had* a beach enclave); there'd be mass rejoicing, fireworks, a special Mass at the cathedral. Now, just let Jesse Jackson and family try to move in and you'd have fireworks, all right—cross-shaped, right on the Jacksons' lawn.

As the sun began to set on the eve of the country's 202nd birthday, Spencer and I made our way down to the weatherbeaten beach club building where the bluebloods were gathering for the annual medley of Americana. When the Yalie choir came on, it was as if we had entered a Ralph Lauren ad. I hated the whole golden-haired silver-spooned group on sight, but even more on thought of their advantages. These men my age were groomed from birth for success at the highest levels. Oh, but what risks they undertook, what struggle; for failure meant a humble, miserable life of cocktail parties and golf. At least the certainty that, spoiled beyond belief throughout childhood, many of their lives would end in tragic, *Dynasty*-size scandal was some consolation.

The rest of Spencer's family drove up the hill to the Hyannisport

Club in the Forrests' antique, seafoam green limousine; Spencer and I went on foot, passing the Shrivers' house, which was about the size of the Grand Hotel on Mackinac Island, doubtless to accommodate a constant Kennedy overflow. While walking through the club's parking lot, Spencer clued me in on the possibility of a glimpse of Jackie O., who supposedly jogged the golf course at sunset. I said I supposed Queen Elizabeth would be following right behind — although by this point even that wouldn't have surprised me entirely. (Does one curtsy, or kiss the royal Reeboks?)

Sure enough, almost as soon as we spoke Mrs. Onassis came trotting our way, wearing a scarf and her trademark shades (more a giveaway than a disguise); she was drenched in sweat (greatest revelation of all — Jackie O. sweats!) and as slim as when America first saw a First Lady dressed in French haute couture. Even from a distance and in running shorts and tennis shoes, she still personified *style*. The shades and broad, high cheekbones created a Garbo-like mystique. "Mystique," that certain cool, aloof *je ne sais quoi*, was what Manfred often said makes people seek you, court you, *want* you. But je ne savais *pas* quoi — I didn't really *understand* it — until now. Of course, understanding it was not the same as achieving it. *That* was not a science, perhaps not even an art — perhaps only an accident of birth.

As she passed us, the great O. spoke. (She didn't seem to know or care that her speaking would leave me speechless for days.) All she said was, "Hi, Spencer." But it was enough.

"Jimmy, put your eyes back in your head or you'll lose them."

"But, Spencer, that was . . ."

"I know, Jackie O. Didn't I tell you we might see her? She's just simple folk. Pay her no mind. She's harmless. She don't bite," he added to tease the "hique" from Dubuque.

It didn't much matter that the Jackie Mystique had left me speechless, for as the Forrests' tasteful, elevated dinner conversation flew overhead from art to politics, I did not have much to contribute. Actually, I thought it best to keep my mouth shut to avoid embarrassing Spencer and blowing my Ivy League imposture with some glaring faux pas. Even so, Spencer was no doubt asking himself how long my charade as a Lake Forest prep could hold up under Miles' withering questioning. He excused us, and we hopped into his VW

Thing and drove off for a night of fun and frivolity in Province-town — the easternmost haven in the United States for Bohemians, artists, and homosexuals.

As we headed down the lonely cape stretch, the fog once again engulfed us. The long, low moan of foghorns seemed to mourn centuries of souls lost to storms at sea, or to the struggle for art, or to unrequited love. Or lust. Perhaps the deacon was out tonight. It seemed a big day for elusive celebrities. I rolled down the window to let fresh air in and morbid fantasies out, and thought instead of Flamingo, Studio, and the pleasant fantasies whose fulfillment might await me upon my return to the city. Finally the soft glow of Provincetown became visible. We pulled in to the Brigadoon-like hamlet and Spencer parked in front of a storybook-perfect "salt-box" building. From inside, slurred, boisterous voices rang out in near-tune with a piano pounding out rough approximations of venerable old show tunes.

"Oh, great. Who hangs out here, Lloyd's and Harc's fathers?"

"Now, Jimmy, there's plenty of variety down there. I thought we might start the evening with something a little nostalgic."

"Nostalgic? I know I'm aging fast at the rate I'm going and all that, but this is stuff the crew of the Pequod could have sung along with." The deacon, for that matter.

As we walked through the door, the music stopped. The clientele was long in the tooth, all right — the better to eat us with, it seemed: At the prospect of a roll in the hay with a smooth, taught young body, dentures dropped and pacemakers shifted into overdrive; like vultures over a dead carcass, they circled, then approached one by one, with touchy-feely introductions, adjusting an ascot here, smoothing back a receding hairline there, popping Tic Tacs into their mouths. One déjà vu per day is enough; but this was Harc and Lloyd revisited, only multiplied in number and pathos. A portly, double-chinned, walrus-like Lothario, stuffed into a seam-bursting brass-buttoned club jacket, approached and cupped his hand around my buttocks. I lost control, and pushed the man barroom-brawl-style into the crowd, drenching him and his fellow lechers with their drinks.

The group cowered in a corner, awaiting my next move, looking frightened and at the same time, I thought, excited by my violence.

I said, "Spencer, I can't take these old faggots. Get me out of here."

Spencer was open-mouthed in shock, but far from pretending he wasn't simultaneously thrilled, he lifted his glass in a toast: "Here's to Midwestern machismo!"

It is one of the most treasured moments of my life, for it was the first time I stood up for myself like a man. I, who as a youth was tortured and taunted as a sissy by my peers for my late puberty, my singing soprano in the church choir, my playing hopscotch with the girls—I had now displayed physical force; I had intimidated other men. I delighted in this sudden revelation of my masculinity. The fly had become the flyswatter. I had finally planted my flag on the Everest of male pride. (We macho men mix our metaphors. Got a problem?)

Leaving the scene of the triumph, we walked down a cobblestone street by the harbor to a wharfside club intriguingly named the Back Room. Though nestled among shipping warehouses and buildings for cold storage of fish, Spencer assured me that this place would have a much younger, livelier crowd.

Right on cue, two leather-clad S&M-outfitted clones, about as clean as though they had just climbed out of the La Brea tarpits, stumbled out the door, one holding the other up as his dinner and nightly tanker load of beer played a return engagement on the cobblestones at my feet. Oh, good—a younger, livelier crowd. The scene inside resembled Picasso's *Guernica*. A tableau of assorted freaks did their unbridled best to live down lifetimes of frustration and persecution: Midget lesbians in skintight denims hugged each other; rail-thin would-be models and transvestites dreaming they were dancers in *A Chorus Line* twirled in a flurry of upturned collars and sequins, checking themselves in the mirrored wall with each revolution for running mascara and out-of-place hair.

Younger, certainly. But if this was Spencer's idea of "livelier," I preferred a nice séance with the ever-effervescent deacon, or some more of Mr. Forrest's charming interrogations. Spencer noticed my displeasure—the gritted teeth and clenched fists may have been the giveaway—and merely shrugged, "You win some, you lose some."

"Well, let's lose these freaks *now*." As we stumbled back over the cobblestones and through the blowing mist to the car, the fog-horn seemed to be no longer mourning but laughing at us. And I may have also heard the deacon joining in. But it could just have been Spencer, giggling at my discomfiture. His laugh is a lot like the deacon's.

The next day we took our leave of the Forrests' American dream. As we passed the barricade and its dozing guard, I took one last look around for John John. All I saw were lingering visions of the previous night's freak show. God, how I detested them all. Was I to be identified as one of *them*? Aside from Bud and Scott, the homosexuals I had bedded were mostly waiters, models, airline stewards and hustlers. On these I was spending my long-pent-up sexual energy, in a continuum of orgasms, a frantic effort to make up for lost time. A seemingly endless array of beautiful male specimens were available by a mere wink of an eye or flash of a smile; and I was as addicted as I'd been to sweets as a child. It was as if the songs "Addicted to Love" and "So Many Men, So Little Time" were composed especially for me. But the scene at the Back Room was a sneak preview of what all my parents' hopes and dreams for their golden boy might come to if I continued on this track. What a slap in the face in return for my father's irreplaceable gift of balls and guts and my mother's doting love and salutary discipline of yardsticks and wooden spoons broken over my (fat) behind. I was beginning to think it might be time to stop smelling the roses before I got stuck by the thorns. I could only wonder if Spencer had deliberately shown me the carnival of lost souls—the sick leatherman, the silly dance queens, the aging, lonely men desperate to turn back the clocks of their lives—in order to demonstrate that too much, too soon might result in too little, too late. The deacon hadn't turned up, but it was as though Dickens' Ghost of Christmas Yet To Come had.

Chapter 7

Rubbing Elbows with the Rich and Famous

A highbrow is the kind of person who looks at a sausage and thinks of Picasso.

— Alan Patrick Herbert

The sobering premonitions at the Cape didn't deter me, once back at 970 Park, from making a beeline to see what new treats and temptations might await on Spencer's answering machine. I found it run to the end, and almost all of the messages were for me. Hitting that playback button was like hitting the jackpot on a slot machine: Out poured a cascade of bewitching new voices, names, invitations. It was wonderful — yet disconcerting. Had I, in cocaine delirium, given the number to the entire male half of the Manhattan telephone book? Or was this the work of a prankster — perhaps one operating out of the Hyannis cemetery? *Would* a ghost leave graffiti saying "For a good time, call Jimmy at. . . ."?

I returned Walter's call first, only because it mentioned tickets to another charity gala. This one sounded like my ticket to stardom. It was, ironically, a Kennedy-sponsored event, benefitting the Special Olympics, the family's pet charity in tribute to Rose's mentally retarded daughter. It was to be the world premier of *Superman*, the movie of the year, at Broadway's Shubert Theater. A concerted media blitz had promoted the film for months. The glitterati would be out in full regalia, knowing full well that the social columnists too would be out in force, their acid-filled pens ready to praise the best-dressed and rip into the worst. Competition would be vicious. Would the winner be Nan Kempner in Halston black taffeta? Betsy Bloomingdale in crepe de chine by Blass? Chessy Raynor in sequined red Valentino? One's face would be met with cordial greetings and clenched-teeth smiles, while one's back received such sweet endearments as "She looks like a gunnysack full of potatoes in that thing," "A bag lady could have done better," and "I suppose pulling her hair tight in that bun is cheaper than a face-lift." "Special Olympics" indeed: the fake smile marathon; the 20-meter back stab; the 24-carat diamond ring flash.

In order to avoid a weekend invasion of "bridge and tunnel" gawkers, the opening was held midweek. I was pacing the lobby of 970 Park like a pendulum on a grandfather clock, waiting for Walter, the doorman eyeing me coldly. Walter's limo finally pulled up to the curbside. The doorman opened the door of the stretch, no doubt anticipating a substantial tip from the limo passenger. What he got was Walter greeting me with his shrillest, campiest "Fabulous, dahling, you look simply faaaaabuuuuulous."

Now the doorman glared at me with hatred. "I would suggest you clean up your act immediately, Mr. Melson, or your host Mr. Forrest's stay in this building will be short lived."

My embarrassment at Walter's flamboyance turned to rage at the doorman's gall. "Enough of your snide looks and comments, white trash. Careful or Mr. Forrest will have you back on your old garbage route where they found you."

"Consider the source, you goddamned dirty hustler."

Walter was rolling in his seat in belly laughter, gasping for air and trying not to spill the coke vial he held in one hand and the Dom Perignon in the other. The doorman's remarks and this glimpse into Walter's self-destructive decadence had me wondering anew about my new-found life in the fast lane. If I couldn't pull the rich kid act off on a doorman, how could I possibly think I could mask the brand of Dubuque from high society? Would the socialites' whispers be about each other, or would they be speculating about how much I was charging Walter for my sexual favors? Did I look like one of those boys leaning against the lampposts on 53rd Street, parading their wares to rich old men from Beekman Place as they slowly passed by in smoked-glassed limos doing their evening "shopping?" Why couldn't *I* have been born a Kennedy or a Forrest? Why couldn't *I* shift effortlessly from one language into another? How does one create a model of urbane sophistication from raw material hardened in a Midwestern mold for twenty years? Who did I think I was, Eliza Doolittle? Like the rain in Spain, perhaps I should have stayed on the plain.

"Walter, tell the chauffeur to turn around. I have nothing in common with these highbrows. They'll chew me up and spit me out and act like I have no right to exist, just like Spencer's dad did at the Cape. I may be a greenhorn, but I have some pride."

"Jimmy, the zirconia queens at this thing have about as much dignity as I do in my prick. Their airs are as pretentious as their art collections. Take away the makeup and girdles and you wouldn't be able to tell them apart from bag ladies. You'll probably be the most real person there."

"Walter, my ancestors didn't come over on the Mayflower and my only trust fund is a thousand-dollar U.S. Savings Bond given me on my high school graduation."

"Forget it, Jimmy, you're trashed before they even see you, whether you're Dolly Parton or Pope John."

We turned the corner of 46th and Seventh. Police barricades had blocked off the intersection to all but "invitation only"-stickered limousines, which were lined up around the block, longer than the Friday night takeoff line at O'Hare. Revolving klieg lights outside the theater were morbid reminders of the ghostly fog lights at the Cape — and its other ghostly presence. Was I next in line for the gallows? "James Melson, you have been found guilty of impersonating a Somebody. . . ." But the teeming crowd of stargazers and paparazzi quickly dissipated my fears. The mere sight of them trying to catch a sight of *me* made me *feel* like a "somebody." Anyway, none of them was holding a noose.

As we inched up to the roped-off entrance, Walter produced two pairs of Porsche Carrera sunglasses, one of which he handed to me.

"Walter, it's eight o'clock at night, what the hell do we need sunglasses for?"

"First of all, they create a mystique. Movie stars wear sunglasses to remain incognito, but really they attract more attention than they divert. Secondly, you don't want to be watching Christopher Reeve through blue dots. And thirdly, the last thing you want is to be caught with squinty eyes in the tabloids."

Walter, his ego practically spilling out the doors, flicked on the light of the vanity mirror to put the finishing touches on his movie-star look. (With his strawberry-blond hair and pale, freckled complexion, he was as convincing as Opie Taylor impersonating Cary Grant.) Outside, the celebrity seekers were readying their autograph books and cameras, and the squealing, nubile teenagers were applying last-minute lip gloss and wetting their panties in anticipation of—whom? Jim Melson and Walter Montfort . . . and of course, Christopher Reeve, whose sight would be enough to take home to their Donny Osmond-postered rooms and weave into dream fantasies of romance with Superman.

A handlebar-mustachioed bouncer opened the car door, and I stepped out onto the red-carpeted sidewalk first. Giddy squeals turned to groans of disappointment. In an instant my bubble of social grandeur had popped. In its place, insecurity rearose like a chronic herpes blister. It was the groans and jeers of my youth all over again. I was a legend in my own . . . limo (and not even my own). So this was how much looks counted for; a vastly inflated currency—a ruble, a rupee, a peso—in the economics of fame.

We entered the gilded rococo lobby. I returned Walter's sunglasses. "Just what kind of mystique were we supposed to create, Walter? From the sound of that crowd I'd say we were about as charismatic as Charles Manson and Lee Harvey Oswald."

"Jimmy, you'd have to be wearing blue tights and a red cape to draw any serious attention tonight." And indeed, since Reeve had left his Superman togs in his closet in favor of a tux, it was his ravishing co-star, Valerie Perrine, who stole the (fashion) show with comic-book-inspired couture: When she arrived, not in the usual black taffeta with conservative neckline, but in a skin-tight suit of spandex—bulging every bit as superheroically as, albeit totally differently from, Superman—all the fashion columnists from *Vogue* and *Mademoiselle* to the *New York Post* and *National Enquirer* broke into delirious applause, the men in the audience into lascivious drooling, and their wives into cold sweats of sheer, jealous hatred.

As the lights dimmed, a horsy-looking woman appeared on stage.

"Walter, who is that old nag?"

"Why Jimmy, you just spent the weekend at her house at the Cape."

"Good lord, Jean Kennedy?"

"Seems to have inherited the masculine Kennedy genes. Probably wears a jock strap under all that taffeta. Rumor has it she couldn't compete on the football field with her brothers, so she had a sex change operation."

"No!" In my naiveté, Walter could have told me she was a reincarnation of Gunga Din and I would have believed him.

Jean thanked the well- and high-heeled patrons for their $500-a-ticket tax write-offs and introduced members of the Kennedys' extended family clan, occupying most of the first ten rows. At last the movie began. I had looked forward eagerly to the sight of Christopher Reeve's basket. I was disappointed. No doubt with a view to preserving the movie's 'G' rating, little supercrotch was in evidence; a combination of costume design, camera angles and cutting-room scissors had unmanned Superman as effectively as a kryptonite jockstrap. As for his relationship with Lois Lane, for all their eroticism they might as well have been Ken and Barbie. (And if *straight* superhero sexuality is taboo, is it any wonder the Boy Wonder was omitted from the recent movie, *Batman*?)

After the movie an announcement was made that guests should remain seated, as limos would be lined up outside according to the row numbers in the theater. Egress would be in graduation ceremony fashion: first the movie stars, followed by the Kennedys, then top-ranking political and corporate chieftains, social register types, and finally other luminaries who, despite their notoriety, had not made the cut for the after-show sit-down dinner at Xenon (54's chief rival for disco supremacy). Needless to say, except for the ushers and janitorial staff, Walter and I were last to exit the theater.

In the limo Walter pulled out his ever-present vial of coke for the four-block ride to Xenon, which due to the limo congestion turned into a forty-minute drive.

"Walter, why don't we just get out and walk?"

"Jimmy, this is a town where the entrance is half the show, and alone worth the price of the ticket. The rush you get from stepping out of a limo in style is like . . . great coke. Speaking of which, care for a nasal refreshment?"

"Aren't you afraid those 'nasal refreshments' are going to eat a big hole in your nose, not to mention making Swiss cheese out of your brain?"

"Does this aquiline work of art look the least bit damaged?" He turned to display his admittedly classical contour.

"It's a masterpiece, Walter, but it's your septum I'm worried about."

"If the septum goes there's always plastic surgery."

"That might be true, but I sincerely doubt a plastic brain would be of much use."

"All that stuff is a bunch of bullshit. The only reason people say that is because they can't afford a hundred dollars a gram. Don't listen to them, dahling. Besides, even if it was true, I've always said 'Live while you can before you can't do any living.' The last thing I'd want is to be eighty, wrinkled and lonely in a nursing home rocking chair listening to Frank Sinatra's 'The September of My Years,' wondering how life could have passed by without my having lived it. I don't know about you but I'd rather be forty dancing my way to an early grave on the ultimate coke high, and if I'm not mistaken, you'd choose that as well. Think of life as a sponge. Soak up as much as you can while you're still well shaped and elastic, and squeeze out every last drop before you've dried up and hardened into a useless, shrunken scrap. Remember that. And now, join me in my indulgence." So I did. Well, such eloquence, such existentialism, such conviction . . . he just stole my nose away.

One snort, four seconds, and twenty-five dollars later, my eyes were bugging out and my tongue was stuck to my palate. Speech poured out unaided by thought, yet every word seemed profound. Suddenly I felt invincible. Celebrities, billionaires, rocket scientists held no terror. I would sweep all before me. "Fear" was a mere sound. My words were spears—no, lightning bolts! How could poor, undersized Christopher Reeve possibly compete? What could Superman do against the Viking god of thunder?

I stepped from the car, momentarily mistaking the rumble of a subway for the earth trembling beneath my feet. Musclebound behemoths (mere mortals) dressed for the occasion in superhero costumes waited to open limo doors and escort guests to their dinner tables. One especially handsome hero approached. "Mr. Montfort, Mr. Cavett, please come with me, I'll show you to your table."

I thought for a moment. "Cavett" was not my human name, I was quite sure.

"Walter, what's this 'Mr. Cavett' business?"

"You've got a comp ticket. Cavett called and couldn't make it so you are a celebrity for the evening. Congratulations."

Omnipotent as I was, changing my visible form was not among my powers. "Walter, I look about as much like Dick Cavett as you do like Sophia Loren."

On cue, Walter sucked in his cheeks. "Grazie, bella bambino, bellissimo. Not to worry, no one's going to be checking the place-cards. If you're nervous about it, casually drop the card on the floor and leave it there." Walter, the operater extraordinaire, had more fancy moves in his tongue than Houdini had in his hands. Walter could challenge the six-time U.S. bullshitting champ Gabe Reynolds for the title.

We proceeded to our table where, as we were among the last to arrive, the others were already seated and on their second cocktails. There it was — a gilt-embossed *Mr. Dick Cavett* place card, proclaiming my guilt, screaming "impostor." And if *it* didn't, then the person to my right surely would, for I'd been put next to Pat Buckley, ubiquitous society page fixture and wife of the ultraconservative writer and commentator William F. Even with a numb nose, I could smell trouble. As I sat down, she raised her eyebrows under her cotton candy bouffant hairdo, then, carefully so as not to stretch her twenty thousand dollars worth of lifted everything, she smiled, "Excuse me, but as you can see that seat is reserved for Mr. Cavett."

For a Viking thunder god, I was, I confess, intimidated. But not Walter the Wizard: he simply took out a pen, crossed out *Mr. Dick Cavett*, wrote in *Mr. James Melson*, and said, "Sorry, Pat, Dick couldn't make it. Had some dreadful interview scheduled with some Nobel Prize laureate. But I know Jimmy well and I'm sure he'll provide you with scintillating dinner conversation."

Thank you, Walter. I mean, if I couldn't entertain Mrs. William F. Buckley with the erudition and wit to which she was accustomed, then my name wasn't Dick Cavett. Once again, I was as out of place as Aretha Franklin at a D.A.R. tea. I sat through dinner trying at least to emulate the others' table manners and pondering the absurdity of existence—mine, in this place. Of my "scintillating" conversation with Mrs. Buckley, nothing need be said, for nothing was. After dinner everyone repaired to the reception area for drinks and other sorts of snorts, while the superheroes cleared away tables to prepare the floor for dancing.

Walter the shmooze artist was immediately off on his rounds: cooing over matrons' gowns, designers' fall lines, models' and actors' looks and social climbers' namedrops; gossiping about who had checked into drug re-hab centers or won a major divorce settlement, and which titled but penniless aristocrat had married into which pennied but titleless family.

I found myself standing alone and helpless in a corner, watching wistfully when a music industry mogul approached with Eileen Ford's numero uno model Jon Murray, the personification of American good looks. Jon stared at me, mesmerizing me with deep-set azure eyes. Walter, never missing a thing, said out of the side of his mouth, "Do I detect a tryst coming on?"

"Now, Walter. What would make you say a thing like that?"

"Just hold onto your heart, Jimmy. On the surface Jon may be a fetching lovemate, but underneath he's the queen of the Continental Baths. You wouldn't believe the stories. Jon epitomizes the word 'sleaze.' Definitely not a homebody. He'll use you like toilet paper and you'll be the one with shit on your face."

At this point, it was so clear that everyone was out to out-trash each other that I figured Walter was just joining in the fun. To me Jon represented a potentially historic coup. I approached him awkwardly and introduced myself; afraid as usual that my Iowa naiveté would come shining through my paper-thin New York sophistication, I once again omitted the annoying little S from my name.

"Oh, Pittsburgh banking family?"

"Uhmm, you got it," I blurted. Spencer's and Walter's lessons must have been sinking in. Develop the mystique. Keep the fantasy alive. Why *shouldn't* I be something more than blond hair and blue eyes? Why *shouldn't* I attract the best of the beautiful, rich and famous?

"Just how much do you have?" Jon inquired.

"Well, Jon, I'm not my father's accountant, but I . . ."

"Not money, bozo — how much do you have between your legs?"

This from a clean-cut, tuxedo-clad fashion plate? Shocking. But I mustn't show it. "Plenty," I shot back. My face flushed and my heart pounded like a Swahili drum. My mouth would have gone dry except it already was Sahara-like from Walter's coke. Jon kept up the hypnotic gaze.

"You ready to get outta this dump, young prince of Pittsburgh?"

Dull duke of Dubuque was more like it, but for this night I would be a scion of old money. Come what may, this most coveted of sex partners would be mine. God, how I wished I had a videocam to tape it and send copies to Scott and Bud! We slipped out the door to a waiting limo and were whisked to Jon's apartment at 405 East 58th Street, otherwise known as "four out of five" (i.e., four out of five residents gay).

The doorman greeted Jon with deference and a conspirational, no doubt nightly, wink at his "catch." I wished he would go give Spencer's doorman lessons. We passed through handsome, gothic-arched, corridors to Jon's studio, furnished in Donghia greys, Le Corbusier chairs and black lacquer wall units displaying a collection of Lalique crystal. Obviously a gentleman of impeccable taste.

Jon dimmed the lights and flipped on a David Bowie record. I lay on his black-suede-covered bed until he emerged from the bathroom, loosening a silk robe to reveal a perfect, sculpted torso.

"Do you like what you see?"

"I love what I see. Show me more."

"Beg me for more. Worship me for more."

Suddenly he reached into his bedside drawer and took out a veritable laboratory of sexual paraphernalia. He handed me a black leather, silver-studded harness. "Put this on," he demanded, and began to grease up a huge dildo with a can of Crisco.

"Jon, I really don't know what you're planning on doing with those things, but whatever it is, it will have to be with someone else. As far as toys go, I'm afraid I'll stick with hula hoops and Tonka trucks."

"Ooooh, sounds kinky. Come on, you chicken shit. Live a little, learn a little. You fucking cock tease. Every stud in this city would give his eyetooth to have a go with me. Looks like I wasted my night on a prissy. Vamoose, muchacho. Hasta luego. Auf Wiedersehen. Interpretation: get the fuck outta here.''

The party was over before it began. That this icon of American physical perfection could have masked such depravity was incredible. Devastated again at falling victim to the myth of the male model, I quickly gathered my strewn tuxedo and, in semi-deshabille, gingerly made my way past the doorman, now slumped and snoring in an armchair.

Heavy rain was now pummeling the canopy, and no cabs were in sight, so I hoofed it the twenty-some blocks back to Spencer's. As I crept into the lobby, drenched, looking like a sewer rat, the doorman gruffly informed me what a mess I was making on his floor, to which I offered the suggestion that he lick it up. So ended my evening of champagne dreams and caviar wishes: in Boone's Farm and sardines.

Nevertheless, the following morning I scoured Spencer's den for stationery; it was time to brag about my life in New York. Three carefully edited versions would be composed: the first for Chicago friends — a steamy account of the previous evening's sex; the second for classmates, highlighting the evening's glamour and my numerous social triumphs; and the third to my parents, reporting on the progress of my independent study on loft space development as a housing alternative in cramped urban settings. This would leave the first group seething with jealousy over my sexual conquests and the second over my membership in elite society, while my parents would be reassured that I had not fallen in with the wrong people. The top drawer of Spencer's burled walnut desk finally yielded a Tiffany box full of eggshell white stationery embossed in gold. Bingo! *That* ought to say what I wanted louder and clearer than what I wrote on it.

I was in the full flight of literary invention when a deafening door slam and a shattering of glass sounded from Spencer's foyer. Unwilling to die at the hands of a drug-crazed, knife-wielding maniac before I'd finished my goddamn letters, I armed myself with Spencer's tennis racket and tiptoed down the service hall. The parquet floor was covered with broken glass and the remains of an English hunting print. In the midst of the carnage was a Hartman suit bag and a monogrammed briefcase. Relieved at this evidence of Spencer's roommate's return, but perplexed at the temper tantrum, I inched my way toward Bob's bedroom door. He was yelling into the phone.

"Goddamn, fucking J. Walter. Their presentation wasn't worth a pile of shit, and L'Oreal gave it to them. And do you know why? Because their fucking account rep has been cunt sucking on their EVP nightly."

I loved the crisp, technical language of business. So Bob had lost a major ad account. Now I remembered Spencer's warning about not crossing Bob. I didn't want to provoke his laying waste any more of the apartment, so I quietly shuffled back to my room and hid from view the remainder of the afternoon.

Early that evening, a loud knock awoke me from a nap.

"Who is it?"

"You know damn well who it is! Let me in, I want to talk to you."

Terrified at his tone, I opened the door to an irate Bob.

"Who the fuck gave you permission to use my Tiffany stationery?" barked Bob.

"Tiffany? But it's just white paper."

"Yeah, at five dollars a pop. Listen, sleazebag, you had better clean up your act or you'll be out on the street hooking your wares with the dregs on 53rd and Third."

The following morning, the shit hit the fan. A registered letter arrived giving Spencer and Bob notice of eviction, citing an institutional-size laundry list of lease violations, the majority concerning the illegal occupancy of a Mr. James Melson and his shameful comings and goings. Bob, beet red, his neck veins popping, his eyes bugging out, instantly marched into my room and proceeded to stuff my belongings into plastic trash bags and deposit them at the elevator door.

Devastated at having cost Spencer his option to buy the apartment for half its market value, I tucked my disgraced tail between my legs and lugged the trash bags out past the triumphant doorman.

"Looks like you're the garbageman, dickface! You try coming back in here and you'll find yourself sitting in the back of a squad car. Get the fuck out of here, jailbait!'' He did have the edge on me, I had to admit.

Ms. Gabor had most certainly *not* sung "Dahling I love you but give me the West Side 'Y'' ''; but that is what it had come down to. I hailed a cabdriver who eyed the bags suspiciously, plainly expecting to end up charged as an accessory to a Park Avenue heist. Throughout the trip across the park he kept a white-knuckled grip on the steering wheel and his eyes on the rearview mirror. Perhaps he thought I was going to pull out a forty-five. If I had, it wouldn't have been to use on him. I sat contemplating my fall from grace and my dismal future, and felt myself sinking into despair.

The cab pulled up to the looming ''Y'' building on West 68th. As I hauled the trash bags into the lobby, the desk clerk gave me a look only slightly less unfriendly than Spencer's doorman.

"I'd like a room, sir."

With an air befitting the manager of the Plaza Hotel, he showed me to a tiny, dingy room bathed in red neon light from the sign right outside the window.

Dahling I love you but get me the hell out of here!

It was now safe to say, with absolutely no risk of error or exaggeration, that James Melson had sunk as low on the ladder of New York life as he cared to sink. I'd had it.

But then, suddenly, I *had* it — inspiration, like a red neon light switching on over my head: What would be more perfect for me, at this point, than a small, friendly, picturesque, Scandinavian college in rural Minnesota?

Chapter 8

The Model Student

Happiness is not a thing you experience but something you remember.

— Oscar Levant

The next day I dialed St. Olaf from a pay phone, with my available fingers crossed, praying that the deadline for registration hadn't passed. A nasally Norske voice answered and informed me it was two days away. Hallelujah. I would not after all have to beg for food in the Bowery, or hook on the meat market of East 53rd — or *cut* meat at the Pack. I would return to school bathed in the glow of New York; my colleagues would crowd around begging for celebrity gossip and tales of Studio 54; and come Christmas, I would land at Dubuque Airport in the epitome of mid-seventies fashion — silver-tipped cowboy boots, bolero tie and western shirt. If I'd hit bottom in New York, I could still skyrocket to the top in and around Northfield, Minnesota.

And so, in September 1978 I was back at St. Olaf. Strangely, there was no welcoming party or press reception. The student body was the same corny old collection of clogs, Icelandic sweaters and Noxema-scrubbed faces that I had left a year before. But at least there was my new roommate, Lon Larson. Lon looked like a male Candice Bergen. The son of a prominent Twin Cities businessman, Lon enjoyed carte blanche at the Ralph Lauren Polo, Clinique and Gucci departments at Dayton's department store. Lon seemed ecstatic at the prospect of living with someone so hip, so chic, so worldly. He was just what I needed: someone who would appreciate — be dazzled by — *die of envy* at — my stories of Studio, limo and cocaine; he would feed the bonfire of my vanity.

Early in the semester I was on one of my nights out with the boys, drinking Heineken and chomping peanuts at the Haberdashery in Minneapolis. I noticed a middle-aged man with long red hair and a beard snapping pictures of me from across the room. What kind of voyeur could this be? I didn't know whether to feel flattered or unnerved. After what seemed like about two rolls of film he approached and offered me his card. I figured he was about to proposition me for some porno publication, or was just some crazed pervert wanting to get into my pants. He introduced himself as Pavlov Jacusak, a photographer, and proceeded to tell me how much "the camera loved" me.

"Do you realize that you personify the all-American boy?"

Never mind that my heritage was 100 percent Danish; I wasn't swallowing any sales pitch, slick or sleazy. I hadn't lived in New York for nothing. I leaned back in my chair and wondered what his next line would be.

"Have you ever considered modeling? You know, you could make a substantial amount of money."

Now this Pavlov had rung the bell and got me salivating. I saw dollar signs flashing, and images of Scott and Bud turning the color of money as they came upon magazine spreads full of pictures of me.

"Why don't you let me set up some test sessions and we'll approach the agencies?"

"You're sure it's not skin flicks you want me for?"

"Do I look like some Hennepin Avenue hustler?"

Actually, he did, but his $2,000 Nikon suggested that he might be something more. I was to meet Pavlov Jacusak at his loft on Nicolet and Tenth the next morning with a varied selection of clothes. Needless to say, sleep did not come easy that night. I hoped I wouldn't show up with circles under my eyes.

One look at Pavlov's loft and my fears evaporated. It was a cavernous, high-tech space with Mies van der Rohe furniture, glass block walls and umbrella lighting. He was legit. As he busily set up for the shoot, I changed into my most chic New York garb.

"No, no, Jim. You're an ingenue. You have to start out with

J. C. Penney before you can graduate to Versace. Here, put these on." He handed me a Van Heusen shirt, double-knit pants and Florsheim shoes.

J. C. Penney. All my New York sophistication, and he wanted to put me in polyester. Reluctantly, I donned the clothes. A stylist placed cardboard inside the shirt and pants to ease out the wrinkles. I felt as graceful as Frankenstein as I shuffled stiffly over to the backdrop.

Pavlov was fussing with the lighting with the intensity of Bertolucci directing an epic. The stylist flipped on a disco beat and the shoot was on. I went into my cliché idea of a modeling pose: sucked-in cheeks, pouting lips, smileless stare . . . even I could tell I looked retarded.

"No, no, Jim. You look like Twiggy. Relax. Be natural. You're selling clothes, not Picasso. Here, smoke some weed and it'll come together."

Suddenly everything came easily. Pavlov was ecstatic.

"Yes, yes. Ten. Perfect. You'll be a star."

The shots were too good to be true. Pavlov immediately messengered them over to Eleanor ("Ellie") Moore, the city's top agency.

"She's going to want to sign an exclusive with you, Jim," Pavlov said. "But don't let her bamboozle you, or she'll control your every move."

Within a half hour, Pavlov's phone rang. It was Ellie.

"James, your test shots were absolutely marvelous. You must come in so we can talk. I can get you work right away."

I soared, elated, to Ellie's office. I had been discovered! How Bud would burn with envy at my being courted by a top agency. My first job was a Dayton's sportswear ad. I was to be at Dayton's photo studio in Nicolet Mall at 10 a.m. sharp the next day.

As I drove up from school the next morning, my eyes were on my reflection in the rearview mirror more than the road. Give them attitude, Jim. You can do it, You'll be fine.

I entered the studio with Pavlov's photos under my arm and my heart in my throat. Would they like me? Was I too fat? Would they notice the cystic acne scar on my cheek? The studio was hopping with flashes going off everywhere, lenses aimed at everything from dining room sets to egg poachers.

"Mr. Melson," Pavlov greeted me. "We're getting ready for your shoot. Please follow Sabrina into the dressing room for your makeup and fitting. We'll see you in the studio in fifteen minutes." Sabrina brought out a baby blue velour jumpsuit. Gag! Bud wouldn't be jealous so much as convulsed in laughter at seeing his ex in some tacky clown suit.

In spite of my big break, as the semester wore on and graduation neared, I plummeted into depression. I was lonely. My classmates had by and large shunned me, and I had had too much of the miseries of gay culture in New York, Chicago and Minneapolis to want to seek out more. What's more, I was bitter about facing another summer in Sundown Town while the rest of my class was being recruited into the corporate brat pack. I decided it best to bear down on my studies and try to improve a sagging grade point average, and take what comfort I could in Haagen Dazs and hopes for my modeling career.

By this point, my "composite" photographs had been distributed far and wide, and jobs began to pick up. Ellie advised me to buy an answering machine. No sooner had I recorded my message than Ellie called with a big assignment.

"Jim, Donaldson's Department Store wants you for a week of shooting for their fall catalogue and a fashion show at the Radisson. There will be a lot of money involved. Can you do it?"

"Ellie," I answered, too excited to be very original, "is the Pope Catholic?"

I crammed for a macroeconomics exam the week before so I could set aside the time for the week of work ahead. I was to meet the photographer, Joel Sebransky, at the Donaldson studios the early part of the following week. Plenty of rest, no booze, and monitoring my caloric intake was of the essence. I had carelessly put on a few pounds in the preceding weeks, so it was au revoir Haagen Dazs, bonjour celery and carrot sticks.

The abstinence must not have agreed with me, because with perfect timing, a hideous cystic zit erupted on my face. I pressed and squeezed the demon frantically, but only made it worse. What I needed was an exorcist. Should I call and say I was sick, or show up looking like a toad and risk rejection? Balls and guts, Jimmy; remember your father's teaching. Stand up to your pimple like a man.

D (Donaldson)-Day arrived and I made my way nervously to the studio. God, please don't let there be fluorescent lights; anything but that merciless all-revealing, zit-enhancing glare.

I walked into a studio flooded with merciless, zit-enhancing glare. I was about to do an about face when a deep voice called out, "Is that you, Jim? Come on in, we're ready for the shoot." I greeted Joel with half my face turned away, then walked sideways with him over to the changing room. I put on the sweats I was to model, then checked myself in the mirror. I felt like Godzilla.

I shuffled out and apologized for my ghastly disfigurement, expecting to be sent on my way, or perhaps sold to a carnival or an institute for scientific research. "Jim, you look fabulous." Joel was humoring me. He was putting me off guard so they could throw a sack over me and tie me up.

"You mean you don't see the zit?"

"Oh, that's nothing. We've got the best stylists in the city. As long as you've got the bone structure, they can work miracles. Trust me, you won't see it in print."

My joy was boundless. My modeling career was saved, my faith in divine providence renewed, my respect for myself as a human being restored, and my zit taught a stern lesson about who was boss. I had come through one of the most severe crises in the life of a model; nothing could stop me now.

A young Japanese stylist went to work covering the pimple with some putty-like stuff. He remarked, "My, what a big one you have there." Perhaps it was the strain of my ordeal, or too many stories about the "casting couch syndrome," but my interpretation of his comment was several feet off. "And just what are you referring to, pervert?" I snapped, sending the poor chap grabbing for his makeup palette and flying from the room.

Yes, my career was progressing—and my prima donnaism right along with it.

More fortunately, so was my income: $75 an hour, $250 a day. I nearly swooned when a $1,250 check appeared in the mail for the week of shooting. *Less* fortunately, so was my spending: a Steuben bowl for my parents' anniversary, a wardrobe to match Lon's, a ski trip to Aspen . . . As for my reviews back home, they were mixed: Mother would save each shot that came out to show her bridge club; Dad, on the other hand, wondered what this faggoty stuff was all about.

I also continued with school, but more and more my "major" was modeling. One day, after a grueling midterm in statistical analysis, I arrived home to find a message from Ellie inquiring about my availability for a Munsingwear shoot. Underwear? I couldn't fathom exposing myself to the world in my skivvies; hardly bridge club show-and-tell material. I called Ellie and told her so.

"You don't have to, Jim. Munsingwear is coming out with a new line of sportswear. You may become the Munsingwear Man if you play your cards right."

A few days later I arrived at Munsingwear's headquarters for a fitting. The chief photographer, was there. The instant I walked in, he and his assistant exchanged a certain lewd, raised-eyebrow smirk that was becoming all too familiar. It was just a matter of how long and how tactfully I could fend them off. Once again, I was fitted for polyesterish clothes I wouldn't be caught dead in. The fitting itself was a touchy-feely free-for-all in which few parts of my body got off lightly. I just gritted my teeth and bore the embarrassing liberties for fear of losing the job. In fact, I even began to play along flirtatiously. What was a bit of fitting room fiddling to the future Munsingwear Man? I was just using a touch of balls and guts, like Dad always told me, only now it was somewhat more literally.

I returned on Monday for the shoot. The paunchy, balding photographer looked as if he had just returned from a makeover at Georgette Klinger, and reeked of Polo cologne. It was clear from the start he was after more than just photos. The way he positioned me for my shots was just short of foreplay. I shuddered. I was getting a pretty good estimate of what the price of future bookings with him might be.

At the end of the shoot, he pulled me aside and asked me to stay for additional shots for his portfolio. Both flattered and suspicious, I agreed. Calm thyself, Jimmy. He just wants you — the future Munsingwear Man — for his portfolio. His *photography* portfolio.

When the remaining staffers had left, he brought out a skimpy swimsuit, a jockstrap, a pair of tattered jeans and a bottle of baby oil. "Excuse me," I spoke up, "but what do you plan on using these photos for, *Blueboy?*"

"Jimmy, my boy, let me assure you, they will not go beyond the confines of my personal portfolio. And *your* portfolio, if you want them. You have a very special sensuality, and I want to capture it."

I bet you do. The fitting room funny business and the heavy-handed posing were one thing (or two), but I was not about to prostitute myself outright for anyone or anything—not *even* becoming the Munsingwear Man.

He told me to lie down on the couch and undo the top buttons of my tattered 501s. Uh oh, here it comes, the grab for the crotch. I unbuttoned the top one. He moved the camera in closer.

"Jim, I need more; unbutton some more." I knew if I did I'd be in trouble, and if I didn't the Munsingwear account would be out the window. But I had to preserve some dignity.

"Two buttons and that's it. And you can forget the jock strap."

"Jim, do you know what you're doing?"

"I think I do. I've had plenty of chances to prostitute myself but I've managed to keep my self-respect, thank you."

Looking embarrassed, he began to put away his equipment (while I closed up mine). "Thank you very much, Mr. Melson," he said curtly, "that will be all." I changed back into my clothes, somewhat in shock, and definitely depressed at how abruptly my bid for the big time had collapsed. No Munsingwear Man. No sweet revenge on Bud and Scott. But I felt proud for not compromising myself; and the prints from the shoot would certainly help my portfolio. Just another life experience, I told myself. And I came out the winner.

And I'll get back at that creep if it's the last thing I do.

I obviously needed to blow off steam—and better sexually than criminally, I reasoned. After a good dinner and a movie, I headed off for the Gay Nineties to pick up the most promising candidate I could find. Just the way that photographer had tried to dominate me, I wanted to dominate someone, someone bigger and stronger than myself—stronger, yet weaker: a steroid-pumped bodybuilder with no brain. And there was the very thing, standing at the bar with a Budweiser in hand and legs wide apart—a mountain of muscle the very sight of whom sent my hormones flowing. A shot of tequila and I was ready to close in.

"What's up?"

"Nothing, how about yourthelf?" I cringed at the lispy response, but was determined to bed him down. He actually offered to show me his etchings (well Erté etchings, but still); I accepted. His name was Bruce. He supported himself as a hairstylist and manicurist. His apartment was decorated in typical 1970s faggotry: Japanese paper wall fans, bird of paradise flowers, and wicker, lots and lots of wicker. Bruce gushed and lisped without cease. I wanted to tape his mouth shut and put a paper bag over his head.

As we undressed, I saw a very small object or organ protruding from his midsection that I soon realized was his penis. I should have known: the old overdeveloped-musculature-as-compensation-for-an-underdeveloped-penis ploy. As he approached with his knobule standing at attention (why it bothered, I don't know), I said "Sorry, I like a little more meat with my meal." Crushed, Bruce crawled off and curled up with his Maltese spaniel for solace.

So I left them, with both their tails between their legs, and crept out of the apartment feeling worse than ever myself, knowing I had literally and figuratively belittled the poor man. How could I have been so insensitive? What a day's work: I'd lost my chance at becoming the Munsingwear Man, and then took it out on some poor, innocent slob.

And the day's tribulations weren't over. I arrived home to find that Lon had moved my bed into the kitchen. It seems he had come across a letter from one of my old tricks in New York, and realized that I was a homosexual. He didn't want anything to do with faggots, he said. This wasn't enough. I later found out that he had also mimeographed the letter and stuck it in the mailboxes of all my friends at the Student Center. It was social genocide. The persecuted fat boy had been resurrected as the persecuted queer. Suddenly all of my friends were no longer available. My depression deepened.

The following week an ad was published in the *Tribune* featuring me in tennis togs. Out of nowhere I was surrounded by giggling sorority girls oohing and aahing as if I had just won an Academy Award. Their boyfriends, meanwhile, took to whistling at me and rating me on a scale of one to ten as if I was a candidate for homecoming queen.

I was a zombie throughout the entire following week. I attended classes but absorbed nothing. Midterm exams were imminent. To make things worse, there was nary a blink on my answering machine. The Munsingwear photographer had probably blackballed me and I would never work again. On one of those bleak afternoons I was poring over incomprehensible equations when Spencer phoned. I thought I'd never hear from him again after getting him evicted; I waited for a torrent of obloquy and hatred.

"Jimmy, I realize you're hardly virgin material but nevertheless, I was wondering if you'd like to accompany me to the Virgin Islands."

"God, Spencer, would I ever, but I really can't afford . . ."

"Stop right there. Do I seem like the type of man who would extend an invitation like that and not pick up the tab?"

I had spring break coming up, and if I couldn't be the Munsingwear Man I could certainly be the Boy from Ipanema. Gratefully and gleefully, I accepted. The first thing that came to mind was what kind of Panama hat to buy. Exactly what was the right fashion statement for luxurious Caneel Bay in St. Johns? Bermuda shorts? Hawaiian shirts? Or the old standby, the revealing Speedo swimsuit?

I was to meet Spencer in three weeks in St. Thomas. Plane tickets would be forwarded to me. I saw the trip as a well-deserved compensation for the loss of my friends, thanks to Lon. I would return a golden god with an island tan. Let my enemies stew in envy and hatred — envy of this ultimate spring break, hatred of me as a homosexual.

Three weeks later I was sitting on the runway of Minneapolis/St. Paul International Airport in a blizzard. The flight to San Juan for a connecting flight to St. Thomas was delayed for two hours. How the hell was I going to deal with an overnight in Puerto Rico? Would Spencer think I had bagged out on him? Finally we took off, and as we passed over Southern Florida the dull blue-grey of the Atlantic became a hypnotic aqua. My God, I was actually getting out of the country, flying off to unimaginable Caribbean fantasies. On board I met a Minnesota Congressman and his wife who were also proceeding to St. Thomas and who volunteered to charter a private plane which would get us in at around 2 a.m.

The chartered plane could well have done double service flying for an international drug cartel, or perhaps a kidnapping ring; the pilot wore army fatigues and unkempt beard. Was I going to St. Thomas or Havana? Would I be met by Spencer, or a gang of machete-wielding terrorists? How would my parents handle a phone call demanding ransom for their son's life? And would they pay?

After endless inner and outer turbulence, we landed and pulled up to the corrugated tin-roofed terminal of the airport in St. Thomas. When I got to Blackbeard's Castle, our quaint little hotel, the light in Spencer's room was still on. He, no doubt, had long since concluded that I had accepted an invitation elsewhere. I opened the door.

"Spencer?"

"Jimmy. Where in the queen's name have you been?" I told him what a nightmare the trip had been.

"Well, I'm glad you finally made it. Let's get some sleep and we'll talk about it over breakfast."

There was one king-sized bed; probably Spencer's idea for how I might repay him for his generosity. He was dreaming. I wasn't going to whore myself, even for this dream vacation.

We awoke the following morning to spectacular sunshine. Lush greenery, tropical flowers — I was in paradise, freed from the arctic grey misery of the Minnesota winter. If on my return Ellie wanted me for a Coppertone commercial, I would be ready.

Our first day's plan was to tour the island. But I had important business to take care of first. As we headed toward the jeep rental I spotted my Panama hat in a chic little boutique, went in and tried on about forty or fifty before finding one that fit. Next stop was at a drugstore to buy Coppertone and Sun In for my hair. The whole object was to return to the Minnesota pasty-facers and flaunt my golden skin and sun-bleached hair. Spencer didn't seem to understand that. He wanted to show me the island. "Jimmy, save the glamour routine for later; let's get on with it." We rented our jeep, and Spencer handed me the keys. Never having driven a clutch car, I jumped into the driver's seat, turned the key, and lurched forward to a dead stop. Spencer was enjoying my klutziness heartily; all the more reason I had to show him my driving prowess. After about four attempts I made it out of first gear and it was clear sailing. As we ascended the mountainous island there were breathtaking views at every hairpin turn. Or so I understand. I, of course, was gripping the wheel for dear life and watching the road ahead in terror.

Two days later we packed up our things and headed to the harbor for our departure to the Caneel Bay resort on St. John's. The ferry looked like the *African Queen*, with a massive, smelly, oily steam engine baking in the sun on the deck. I boarded taking great care not to dirty my sailor whites. The captain pulled a cord and blew an ear-shattering brass steam whistle to signal our departure. I even *felt* like Bogart as we steamed into the Bay—that is, Bogart with a painful sunburn, which forced me to move in slow motion like a creaky geriatric. (I hadn't needed the heavy sunscreen Spencer had offered me; *my* skin was immune from my years of lifeguarding. *I* could manage fine with the baby oil.)

A chauffeur with the darkest skin I'd ever seen brought us from the port into the lush grounds of the Rockefeller resort. Spencer was obviously spending a fortune on our stay in this island paradise. We pulled up to a shuttered, tropical-style house with cypress floors, overstuffed white canvass-covered furniture, and again, a king-sized bed. Spencer must have imagined he was on his honeymoon. We unloaded our luggage and dressed for dinner at the exclusive Bayside Club. The menu had no prices listed; the shock would be all Spencer's. I ordered a Mai Tai, which came with a paper um-brella planted in it, looking like some sort of dessert. Despite my sunburn, I felt like a movie star in my Panama hat and blue blazer. Dehydrated from the heat, I chugged the Mai Tai and immediately ordered another. As I listened to Spencer's campy humor and looked out across the shimmering water of the moonlit harbor and its lights, all I could wish for was that the man sitting across from me was the man of my dreams.

The gold-embossed menus arrived and the selections literally started me salivating. I wanted the lobster, which I'd never had before. The steaming dish arrived with a bewildering battery of tools. How did one penetrate this forbidding red armor? I knew Spencer was watching, waiting to enjoy a laugh at my Iowan inepti-tude; and I was determined to deny him, and to handle the operation as routinely as a Dubuque drive-in hamburger. I chose my weapon: the nutcracker-like thing. I cracked the beast's back. I was instantly blinded. Juice squirted me in the eye, and, to add insult to injury, over the better part of my clothes. This creature *might* have been dead (I'm far from sure); nevertheless it seemed to sense it was up against a beginner, and it meant to press its advantage. If so, it was deceiving itself; for I was angry now, and in fighting trim. Ferociously, I tore off its miserable legs — I can't remember how many, but there were lots — and cracked open its belly. Zip — nothing but guts. Spencer was starting to enjoy the slapstick. Something had to be done, and fast. Even I knew there was meat reputed to be in the claws, so I attacked them next. Bingo! Succulent chunks of steaming meat, doused in melted butter and sweetened with victory.

I got no more nonsense from the lobster that night. And as the second Mai Tai started to kick in, my thoughts turned toward the steel drum band I had heard at a locals' bar down by the harbor. Spencer wanted to return to the room to listen to his organ music tapes. With the king-size bed very much in mind, I asked if he would mind if I headed down to the bar. With luck he would be asleep by time I arrived home.

No such luck. I thought I'd finished with troublesome claws for one day; but when I got back from the bar, as soon as my head hit the pillow I felt Spencer's hand groping for my crotch. Without a word I pushed his hand away, but he persisted, like a fly on a piece of meat. I felt like a flyswatter. "Spencer, stop it!" I finally yelled.

"I'm sorry," he mumbled, embarrassed.

Now *I* lay awake; feeling guilty yet again that I couldn't reciprocate for all Spencer's lavish spending on me. Finally, I had to go to my medicine kit in the bathroom and take some Nyquil so I could get some sleep.

I went snorkeling the next day — paddling around the most beautiful tropical fish tank in the world, feeling like a young Lloyd Bridges. I came out exhilarated and full of energy, and decided to take a run on the beach. I came upon a beautiful-looking couple, one of whom was doing jetés on the sand, his bronzed legs gleaming in the sun. It was a wonder he managed to keep his well-packed pouch under wraps with all that violent flexing and those undulating movements. I complimented him on his talent, and he explained that he was with the American Ballet Theatre and was practicing for the upcoming seasonal tour. His lover was an artist in Soho. I looked at them both and almost cried, jealous of their happiness, wishing that I too could enjoy this paradise with my one and only.

I enjoyed the remaining days of bicycling, hang-gliding, water-skiing and sunning nonetheless, and was sad indeed when it came time to go back to school. But at least there was my tanned and bleached glory to flaunt, and needless to say, I did — strutting around the athletic center, sensuously caressing my bronzed body in the shower, carefully lathering and creaming my skin to prevent it flaking or peeling; I even bought a sunlamp to preserve my precious glow. Further palliating the post-holiday pangs were the beckoning blinks of my answering machine. Ellie, it seemed, wanted me to play a football player in a commercial for Taco Bell. Well, if Taco Bell wasn't a stepping-stone to stardom, what was? Filming was to be in the Edina restaurant and my role was merely to sit in a booth, take a bite, smile, and after the take was cut, spit it out into a bucket to avoid getting sick.

A bite turned into countless bites for countless takes, curing me for life of any appetite for tacos. But for the chance of getting on TV, I would have eaten at every Taco Bell from Green Bay to Guadalajara. Soon they would be calling me for roles in soaps; who knows, maybe a feature film role. (If they needed a starry-eyed dreamer with delusions of grandeur, I knew the part inside out.)

No such chimeras *or* cameras materialized, of course. The year 1979 wore on without much excitement. But its very end brought the end of school and the beginning of a new relationship. When New Year's Eve and graduation approached, I decided to celebrate both — especially my long-longed-for liberation from academia — with a night in Chicago, after which I'd go on to Dubuque. I called an "Ole" (St. Olaf) alum, Lynn Olsen, affectionately known as Yoda for her extraterrestrial intelligence and big ears, to see if she could put me up for the night. Yoda was now a graduate student in sociology at Northwestern University whose ambition was to conquer the massive problems of the Caprini Green public housing project, the notorious 1960s dream-turned-nightmare. This wholesome-looking idealist detested any form of artifice, from makeup to the glamour and glitz of the city, and was perfectly content to curl up in her flannel jammies and down-filled slippers with a cup of camomile tea. Which would not hinder *my* plans in the least.

"Yoda, honey, this is Jimmy. I finally made it . . . by the skin of my teeth, I might add. No tassels and robes, no ceremony, no fanfare, and worst of all, no on-campus interviews. Horrors alive if I had to remain one more semester at that monastery. I need to let loose for some New Year's Eve frivolity and thought I'd come to Chicago to visit and get it all out of my system."

"Sure, Jim, as long as you keep that hyperactive libido of yours under control, i.e., dragging home any New Year's Eve babies will be strictly verboten."

"Please, I may not have much dignity but I do have some sense of propriety." As much as I loved and respected Yoda, she knew as well as I did that I was merely using her apartment as a fall-back in case my New Year's Eve sexual fantasies remained just that.

Finals ended and, jubilant and excited, I flew to Chicago and made my way to Yoda's. She told me that my ex-roommate Lon and Dodo had just left.

"Who or what is Dodo?" I assumed Lon had acquired a dog, or an extinct bird.

"Jim," Yoda said, "I thought you knew. Dodo is Lon's Italian lover."

"That's a strange name for a woman." Yoda, Dodo . . . it was starting to sound like Tolkien.

"Jim, Dodo is a man."

That fucking bastard. I was dumbstruck — although my sixth sense *had* told me Lon was gay when we were roommates. Perhaps "outing" *me* in his barbarous fashion had been his way of testing the waters, to see how other people, friends and associates, reacted. Well, he saw. Friends were friends no more and I was lucky if I could get a nod of acknowledgement. If I'd had the money I would have loved to hire a hit man to *really* "out" Lon.

But no Lon or Toto or Yoyo was going to spoil my evening. My destination was Carol's, Chicago's hottest new gay club. Around ten I strolled into the place, in my silver-tipped cowboy boots, red bandanna head band and dark Ray-Ban sunglasses, doing my best to exude all the glamour of New York and the *hauteur* of an opera diva. There was a show called *Two Tons of Fun*: a pair of enormous black women whose rendition of "It's Raining Men" drove the queens delirious. Old familiar faces dotted the confetti-filled room, some meriting reacquaintance and others to be avoided at all costs. At the bar I noticed a Tom Selleck look-alike, the very embodiment of masculinity. Then he noticed me, and flashed me a brilliant smile. I seemed to have found my New Year's Eve baby.

I'd had barely enough time to find out his name was Keith, he was from Rockford, Illinois, and he was a beer drinker (who had already taken a good deal of it on board), and to tell him that I was in a nine-month hiatus (which was in fact what I was planning) before heading out to USC graduate school in LA — when who did I spot out of the corner of my eye but Bud. Without even thinking, I grabbed Keith and gave him a long, deep French kiss that Bud couldn't possibly miss, and didn't. I looked just in time to see him turn to his friends. It was a moment to cherish. And Keith didn't mind it either. He and I both wanted to pursue the subject further, but were constrained by our overnight accommodations. We exchanged numbers and said we'd talk the following week to arrange a rendezvous in Rockford.

Throughout the 3 1/2-hour drive back to Dubuque next morning, all I could think of was Keith. Was this hot-looking man worth canceling my grad school plans? But what would I do in Dubuque if I stayed? Meat packing was certainly out of the question; as much as I loved pig fetuses, I felt I'd handled my share. Insurance sales? Cleaner, but just as boring. I suddenly felt bitter about my education. What good were my four years of academic misery in pursuit of a liberal arts degree? The only thing that became liberal were my bedtime habits. On the job front, things didn't look sexy at all.

Keith called the following week and invited me to Rockford for the weekend. I was to meet him at Rocky's Love Park Tap. This proved to be a redneck drinking hangout, with a pool table, giant TV screen, bowling trophies lining the bar's back wall, and a clientele that, if they only knew my sexual preference, would undoubtedly have escorted me to the back alley to kick the shit out of me. Suddenly I wondered if my New Year's Eve libations might have affected my judgement about Keith. I imagined him pulling up in a mufflerless, beat-up pickup truck. Meanwhile, however, he was nowhere in sight. I tried to call him from the pay phone; no answer.

I was already leaving, fuming that my perfect date record had been marred by a no-show, when a gleaming black 280Z screeched into the parking lot and out hopped Keith in faded Calvin Klein jeans and red flannel shirt, charmingly flashing his pearly whites and apologizing for my wait.

"I'm starved," he said. "How about you?"

"Do you have to ask? But please, not this sleaze pit. I felt like a guppy in a shark tank in there. Really scary crowd."

"They're harmless for the most part. The only things they care about are pussy, the Cubs, beer and overtime. How 'bout we call Red Lobster for take-out surf and turf?"

We got the dinner and headed to Keith's place. It was the lower half of a putrid green stucco duplex, and was decorated in early *Newlywed Game*. Keith obviously had no interest in the decorative chatchkas found in most urban homosexual digs. Thank God.

My previous engagement with lobster had been like making war; this time it was like making love. Keith and I watched each other as we sensuously sucked the meat out of the claws and legs and tails. As one kind of appetite was sated, another was whetted. Then dessert — two twenty-five-ounce cans of Heineken and two joints. We dimmed the lights, flipped on the theme from *American Gigolo*, and began our courtship dance. With his thick mustache, kissing Keith was like kissing the Fuller Brush man; but his expressive Bambilike brown eyes and full, sensual lips more than made up for any mouth abrasions. Attention to the lips was soon transferred to the growing bulge in his pants. Yes indeed, this man was all there — far beyond my expectations.

We awoke the next morning to six inches of freshly fallen snow, and a serious case of ski fever.

"Come on, Keith, we've simply got to get to Dubuque. Six inches of fresh powder! And I can get us free tickets at Sundown."

"Who do you have pull with, some hot ski instructor?"

For a rare change I decided not to mention my father's part-ownership; I felt sure any bragging would be an instant turnoff. "Oh, just through friends of my folks who have stock in the place."

At a gas stop I told Keith I had to stop at home to pick up my ski gear, and asked him to meet me at the Loft bar on top of the hill. By the time I arrived he had already had a few beers. My casual, modest mentions of my skiing expertise seemed to have intimidated him. (His own scratchless equipment had obviously seen little more than vertical "action" in his closet.)

"Don't worry," I urged, "we've all got to start someplace." I skied down to the end of the bunny slope and watched as after fumbling with his bindings, he wobbled down the hill in a timid snowplow, hit a patch of ice and landed on his rear. "Well, Keith, you may look the part, but I think you should probably stick with the ski bunnies at the bar." What could get a macho man back on his skis faster for another heroic try?

This time, just for variety, he executed a perfect, textbook belly flop into the snow.

Far and away Keith's best moment of the day came after I suggested we call it a day and hit the bar for some Irish coffee in front of the fireplace. The snow bunnies immediately started ogling him, gushing and giggling, hoping no doubt that he'd go over and buy them drinks. Finally, frustrated at his lack of response, an overly made-up blond in white Hansen boots and hot pink ski outfit approached.

"Hi, Handsome. Thought I might introduce myself."

"Don't bother, honey, I like boys. You're wasting your time." Little miss snow pussy called Keith a sick demented pansy and turned away in a huff, leaving two sick demented pansies in barely contained hysterics.

Keith and I decided to meet the following weekend in the historic town of Galena, Illinois, across the river and about twenty miles from Dubuque. In the meantime, I would comb the *Telegraph Herald* employment section for a job. A recession was on, and had hit local employment hard. The construction industry was in a slump, which in turn meant major layoffs at John Deere, and on top of it there was a strike at the Dubuque Packing Company. Unemployment in Dubuque had reached a shocking 20 percent. The only jobs available were for tool and die makers, janitors and auto mechanics. In desperation I decided to try Job Service of Iowa, the quasi-public employment agency of last resort, expecting, at best, exciting career opportunities in garbage pickup, sewer work or highway cleanup. I was surprised to find a listing for Associate Economic Development Planner at the East Central Intergovernmental Association, or ECIA. Quite a mouthful (not that I was averse to the occasional mouthful), and just the sort of thing that would impress my anticorporate, socially conscious ex-classmates. Nevertheless, I applied and soon after was granted an interview with the director, Bill Baum, a would-be politician with salt-and-pepper hair, a handlebar mustache, and the air of a self-styled ladykiller. I shmoozed my way through it quite deftly, thank you (God knows, between Gabe, Walter and Spencer I had to learn something); and the following week a letter came offering me a whopping starting salary of $11,000 a year. Wowee, five figures. Regardless, it was a prestigious title which I could flaunt far and wide. I began immediately by calling Keith, who was considerably more elated by the news than I was.

We met as planned in Galena, and as we drove around the winding streets, admiring the flawlessly preserved limestone miners' cottages and Victorian mansions, I suddenly decided this was where I wanted to live. Keith was equally enthusiastic: the ideal place, about ninety miles from Rockford, to spend weekends with me. We stopped at a real estate office on Main Street. The proprietor proved to be part of Galena's sizeable and highly aesthetics-conscious gay community. He showed us a photo book of the current rental listings, and one called the Osprey Nest caught my eye: an 1840s federal-style brick house that supposedly had once been owned by Ulysses S. Grant's minister. We drove up to look at it. It sat alone at the edge of a cliff overlooking the town. You entered through a wrought iron gate and into the top level, where there was a double parlor with wide-plank pine floors and a marble fireplace. Below was the living room, with a Ben Franklin stove, the bedroom, the kitchen, and a stone grotto whose walls were covered with figures of pixies and wood nymphs painted by a noted local artist, and to which the previous tenant, a well-known children's book author, would bring groups of children for story-telling sessions. Pixies, wood nymphs — why not a couple of fairies?

And now, as they say, the bad news. Although the place's charm was unmatchable, so was its impracticality. Water was gathered in a cistern from rain and snow melt-off from the roof. Pigeon droppings had contaminated the system, and any use of the water, even for brushing teeth, would, as I was to discover, bring on full-scale dysentery. Another minor inconvenience: there was no insulation. In winter, without a fire in the fireplace a glass of water would freeze, and the pipes, of course, would burst. Other little touches included cobwebs and condensation mold covering every surface, general, all-pervasive filth, and a several-month-old roast beef thoughtfully left behind in the refrigerator, which, when opened, filled the whole place with a special, indescribable ambience.

Could I afford to rent a house, even this one, on my paltry salary? I *did* have an alternative: Mother and Dad were leaving to spend the winter in their condo in Naples, Florida, and I could have the run of their house. But I immediately forgot that, and the pigeon droppings, and the roast beef, when we heard the rent. Probably about the same as in Grant's day: $150 a month. Sure, we would have our work cut out for us; but all I saw or cared about now were the *possibilities*. Galena, make way for the newest member of your enclave of decorating-happy fairies!

Three weeks of scrubbing and painting later, Keith and I were meandering down Main Street, combing the antique stores. The first stop was EGK Antiques, a little shop crammed with bric-a-brac and knickknacks and overflowing with eucalyptus, baby's breath and potpourri. The owner introduced himself as Ed.

"My," he cooed, "it's been a blue moon since such a striking couple of men graced my little boutique. What brought you to our charming little hamlet?"

"I just rented the Osprey Nest."

"Oh," he winked, "it's darling; perfect for lovebirds."

Good God, was it so obvious that Keith and I were "together"?

I lowered my voice an octave or so. "Well, Ed, it's been a real pleasure meeting you but there's a Lakers game I want to see. I'm sure we'll see you around." Keith rolled his eyes; he knew full well I'd never watched a basketball game in my life.

"I'm sorry to hear that," Ed said. "I was going to ask you upstairs for a cognac." We thanked him kindly, insisted on a rain check, and, as soon as we were outside, simultaneously burst into laughter.

"Can you believe that nelly old queen?" I said. "What a character. Can't you just see him fussing over his toupee in his boudoir, and struggling with his girdle?"

At the next antique shop window, I fell instantly and completely in love with a superb honey-colored pine wardrobe with molded cornice and hand-carved raised-panel doors. I think I would have traded Keith for it. As it turned out, I couldn't have it without him. When I balked at the $750 price tag, he came to the rescue, wallet in hand, insisting that the place where he spent his weekends had to have it. I could have made love to him *and* the wardrobe then and there. (But that could wait.) It was a token of one beautiful friendship—me and Keith—and the beginning of another: me and antiques. In fact, the quest for new (and old) possessions was to be my chief obsession throughout that year. If I could no longer be "Like a Virgin," I could still become the "Material 'Boy.'"

As though I hadn't had all the joy I deserved for one day, when we arrived home with the wardrobe there was a call from Ellie Moore regarding a week's shooting for an Arctic Cat Snowmobile catalog. They would fly me up to northern Canada at $250 a day. I didn't know how I could get a week off from my job at the ECIA; I'd only been there a few weeks. But Bill, my boss, didn't even call me a flaming faggot and laugh me out of his office as I expected. I flew to Canada, did the shoot, and came back feeling as if I was on a roll, and rolling—relatively—in dough.

Now, to continue the metaphor, my heart was set on new wheels. My trusty old Wimpy was on his last, and ever since seeing the Kennedy brats come screeching into their driveway in a BMW, that had been what I wanted. Keith rolled his eyes at my Kennedy-envy and warned me that a wardrobe was one thing, but a BMW was out. But I had earned enough in Canada for a down payment.

The closest dealer was two hours downriver in Clinton. Keith raced his 280Z down the winding river road at lightning speed.

"Can't you crank this hunk of tin up any faster, Keith?" I teased, picturing him eating my new Beemer's dust. We turned the corner onto Main Street and suddenly, there on the lot sat the car of my dreams, a gleaming white 302i. I jumped out of the car screaming "It's me, it's me, wrap it up."

"Yeah, well you haven't even checked out the sticker price and that will be yours too." Keith had a point. I looked. The price was identical to my annual salary. Father would have a coronary if he knew I was even contemplating this, I thought. It was true—from sardines and Pickett's beer origins I'd gone on to pâté de foie gras and Dom Perignon tastes. And I meant for the banquet to continue — by hook or by crook.

The way the dealer looked down his nose at me, I had an excellent idea where I wanted to tell him to put his BMW. Even ruder was the awakening I got upon hearing the financing payment schedule. I wouldn't be dining on steak and lobster for a while. But I'd live on peanut butter and crackers just to have that piece of machinery sitting outside the Osprey Nest. Two weeks later my credit approval miraculously came through. (Keith said I must have let the dealer give me a blow job.) I had my Beemer!

And what better use for it than to resume my other obsession, antiques? Everything I did now became a treasure hunt. About a week after I got the car, Keith and I drove up to Door County, Wisconsin, a peninsula on Lake Michigan, to go snowmobiling. On the way through Bailey's Harbor we passed a strange little vacant house covered with colorful wood carvings. On top was a carved, five-foot, three-dimensional horse-shaped weathervane. "Stop!" I yelled. "Back up!" We got out to take a closer look. "I've got to have it, Keith," I said. In an adrenalin-powered antiquarian frenzy, I shimmied up a pole at the side of the house to the roof, lifted the vane off its bearings and dropped it to Keith, who was nervously watching for any witnesses of my thievery. I was elated at my folk art coup. I eventually took the piece home to my parents, who thought it was kindling wood for the fireplace. "Dad," I said, "do you realize this is worth thousands?"

His only comment was, "You've got to be off your nut. You couldn't pay anyone to take that rotting piece of wood."

That hurt — but nothing he said could have stopped my antiquarian juggernaut. By the end of the year, when Keith and I decided to take a two-week vacation and drive to Florida, it was the same thing. I insisted it would be more interesting, we would see more of the real America, if we took the back roads instead of the monotonous interstate. By now, of course, Keith had my number: "I know what your scheme is. I'll be doing all the driving and you'll be scouting the countryside for folk art." I got my way. I usually did.

What I got when we got back was less pleasant. I returned to the office (I was still at ECIA) to find a large three-ring binder on my desk, entitled "Guidelines for Developing an Overall Economic Development Plan." This was a plan for economic development in our region, which we had to complete and submit annually to ensure funding for our grant — and thus for my job. Well, here was the economic picture: With interest rates nearing 20 percent, no one was making capital investments; layoffs were at catastrophic levels. Dubuque had an unemployment rate of 21 percent, one of the highest in the country. What could I put in the report? "Our best prospect for economic development would be an expansion of Pickett's Brewery, as thousands of workers seek to drown their unemployment sorrows"?

What's more, rumors ran rampant about the incoming Reagan administration's plans to eliminate government waste. That *had* to mean my job.

Sure enough, not long after Reagan's inauguration the axe fell. What the hell was I going to do now? Move somewhere else, I supposed. But what about Keith? Which was more important to me, a career or my relationship? I really had no choice — I had to make a living. I braced myself and decided to attack New York again. When I told Keith, he flew into a rage, then broke down and cried, pleading with me not to go. I knew just how he felt — pretty much the way I'd felt when Bud had dumped me. And not much worse than I now felt myself.

Chapter 9

My Son, the Banker

The very substance of the ambitious is merely the shadow of a dream.

— William Shakespeare

Ours is a world where people don't know what they want and are willing to go through hell to get it.

— Don Marquis

I knew what I wanted, now that I was back in New York: the ultimate corporate banking job; a title, prestige, money, the whole bit. And I was relentless in my pursuit of it — and oh so realistic: It would be no different, I figured, than BSing my way into Café de Harvey in Chicago.

I sent résumés to every bank in the Yellow Pages, from Ameri-Trust to Bank of Zambia. Weeks went by with no response. Why wasn't my résumé working? True, in reality my planning job had been little more than two years of paper shuffling, dirty joke telling and magazine reading; but with my shrewdness and cunning, I had not mentioned that in the résumé, but had loaded it with such sure-fire catchwords as *spearheaded, developed, liaisoned* and *coordinated.*

One night, Spencer — who I was staying with again in his new place, and who bore no grudge over his eviction — invited me to a small dinner party that he was giving. Also invited was a handsome Southern architect named Jamie Wallace, who was in the talking stages of a co-op loft development on West 23rd in partnership with Spencer and the other dinner guests. As often happens, drink had brought out Jamie's Southern drawl with enough vengeance to re-pay the Civil War.

"It's a mighty fine pleasure to meet you, Jimmy. I've heard lots 'bout you. You look like you're everything Spencer said you wur."

"Jimmy's looking for a banking job here in the city," Spencer explained, "and hasn't been having the best of luck."

"That's a real shame. Whar you from?"

I glanced at Spencer and then to the floor. "Dubuque."

"Dubuque?! Whar the hell is that?"

"Iowa."

"Iowa? Ain't that whar they grow potatas?"

"That's Idaho."

"Oh, yeah. That near Cincinnati?"

"Sorry, that's in Ohio."

"Well shiiit. A smart little guy like you should be gettin' offers from all over. I tell you what, I just designed a ski house in Aspen for George Harris. George is President and CEO of Manufacturers Hanover Leasing Corp. It's the largest leasing company in the world. Why, he's a gol-dang genius, Jimmy. Why don't you give me your résumé and I'll give it to him personally, with a recom-mendation that would make Rockefeller look like a banking green-horn in comparison."

My mouth dropped to the floor. I only hoped *this* wasn't drink speaking, too.

"Are you serious, Jamie?"

"Sure I am. Ol' George's gonna have the most beautiful house in Aspen cuz a me. He owes me one."

I ran instantly to my folder, got ten copies of my résumé and presented them to Jamie.

"Well, well, well. You are quick on the draw. George will ap-preciate that."

I sat through dinner with an ear-to-ear smile.

"Why don't you give me a call on Wednesday? I'll see if I can get in touch with ol' George in the meantime."

"Jamie, if I get a job, I promise I'll take you to dinner anywhere you want."

"You're on. How 'bout Lutece?"

Spencer almost choked on his seven-layer cake. "Better sell your car, Jimmy. Lutece is the *restaurant Français numbre un* in New York. *Très cher*, I warn you. If you get the job, you'll know what Chapter Seven is firsthand before you want to."

I ate, slept and drank George Harris and Manufacturers Hanover until Wednesday morning. At ten Jamie called.

"Jimmy, you got yourself an interview. George's office at 270 Park Avenue, top floor, next Thursday at ten. How 'bout that? Save those pennies 'cause you just may need them for Lutece, and I love good champagne. I just may quit drawin' houses and become a headhunter for unemployed Iowa farm boys. I should let you know something about George. He's a pretty intimidatin' individual. Real serious. Never smiles, never jokes. 'Nuf said, okay?"

The opportunity of a lifetime, I kept saying to myself riding up the elevator the following Thursday. But how will I convince this CEO, this demigod of finance, to choose a B student from a small Midwestern school out of the teeming sea of available Ivy League candidates?

I stepped out at the fiftieth floor into a group of heavyweight (literally and probably figuratively) banking men having a nice, polite meeting: "That dickless sleazebag would screw his mother if he had one," one bawled. "He's got no equity and he's trying to push a guarantee on us from a bunch of ex-cons. Forget it." When I'd entered the huge building I'd felt about three feet tall; now I was down to a foot and a half. But these guys were also a reminder: balls and guts, Jimmy. Balls and guts. You can do it.

An ultra-chic receptionist greeted me from behind an antique Chippendale desk.

"May I help you?"

"Yes, ma'am, I have an appointment to see Mr. Harris. James Melson."

"Mr. Nelson?"

"Melson. M as in Mary." (I was good and tired of "M as in Mary," frankly, and would have preferred Manly, Masculine, or Muscular, but that was a bit weird for people like this receptionist.)

"Please have a seat. I'll tell him you're here."

After a seemingly endless wait of collar and tie straightening and paging absentmindedly through a *Wall Street Journal*, of which I understood about as much as the Torah, I was shown in. Harris, balding, stone-faced, sat behind a bare inch-thick glass table; no mountains of paperwork — not a single sheet.

"It's a great pleasure to meet you, Mr. Harris. I really appreciate the opportunity — "

Harris was in a hurry. "Tell me, Mr. Melson, why do you want to be a banker?"

His brusqueness and stoniness threw me off so that I forgot my whole well-rehearsed speech. I continued *extempore* as well as I could.

"Well, as an economic development planner for the past two years in the Midwest, my job was to write grants to siphon off as much federal money as possible for projects which made no economic sense: infrastructure development and public housing for dying farm communities in a region with over twenty percent unemployment. This was a difficult thing for me to rationalize for myself. I consider banking to be at the root of America's strength, and I want to help make intelligent decisions about the distribution of the country's money. I was discouraged to the point of resignation, Mr. Harris, but Reagan made the decision for me when he took office and eliminated the Economic Development Administration. Frankly, I'm glad he did. Now maybe this country can get back on its feet, clean up the Carter deficit and turn things around."

"Well, Mr. Melson, that's quite an astute answer. Right now, we don't have anything available in leasing, but I'll see what I can do at the bank for a corporate lending job which I'm assuming you'd be interested in. There's a ten- to twelve-month training program. If you make it through that, and only then, you will be a banker. We'll be in touch."

George stood up, extended his hand, and smiled, displaying brownish teeth which gave him a horrifying, demonic look. Now I could understand Jamie's comment about him rarely smiling. But who cared about bad teeth at a moment like this? I could discuss them with him at some future time. Right now, as I rode fifty floors back down, I was smiling ear to ear, thrilled with my impromptu performance. I composed my own reviews: "A tour de force of eloquence." "Patriotic and inspiring." "Fearlessly honest." "Mr. Melson has redefined the job interview." A woman who got on the elevator midway said, "My, you look jolly."

"I am," I answered. "Santa Claus couldn't hold a candle to me today."

Three days later, Harris phoned. This was it. They want me!

"James," he said—you had to love the guy, rotten teeth and all—"James, do you like opera?"

"Opera? To be honest with you, Mr. Harris, I've never been to one."

"Well, then, maybe it's time you should. A friend canceled and I have an extra ticket. How would you like to accompany me?"

"Well, I'd be honored, Mr. Harris." What else was I going to say?

"Good. It's a matinee performance of Wagner's *Parsifal*. Maybe a little heavy for a novice, but the Met is truly superb. Meet me in the cocktail lounge of Alice Tully Hall, Saturday at one. We'll see you then."

That was it. Not a frigging word about the job.

Saturday came and I donned my best opera attire: my interview suit, and a different tie. George I could only imagine arriving wearing a sash and monocle, taking his place in the center box and greeting those below with a clicking of the heels. Meanwhile, his bald head was nowhere in sight. I was beginning to wonder if this whole thing was some sick joke Jamie had dreamed up.

He arrived. No monocle. "James. Welcome to culture. Are we ready?"

He sounded downright laid back, for *him*—like he had let down what little hair he had for this funfest. Which of course turned out to be four torturous hours of wailing. Whatever wag said "Wagner's music isn't as bad as it sounds" was wrong. I sat through it all feigning whatever interest and emotion seemed to be indicated, all the while thinking of Studio 54, hot men, and the beautiful people I had deprived myself of over the past two weeks while preparing for the interview.

Finally, after about 38 curtain calls, George bid me adieu at the door. Still not a word about the interview or the job. Jimmy, you blew it. Frustration. Confusion. I was at the end of my rope: my finances were exhausted; even my résumé supply was exhausted. (My thirst for Wagner was *definitely* exhausted.)

Sunday night, after a much-needed weekend of Wanton abandon to drugs, sex and rock 'n' roll, Jamie called.

"Jimmy, I's claimin' mah reward. You got the job. Lutece here we come."

"What do you mean? I didn't get any job. All I got was *Parsifal*, Acts one through eighty-four."

"Bullshit."

"Exactly."

"I just got off the phone with George. The bank's gonna hire you for their corporate training program."

"Well, why didn't *he* call me? I didn't even get a letter."

"You just check your mailbox tomorrow 'cause there'll be a letter there that's worth about $200 for dinner at you know where. Give me a call when you get it."

Jamie sounded for real, but my bubbles had been burst so many times in the past. And the meaning of the "date" at the opera still baffled me.

Next morning the mailman handed me the usual heap of junk mail, and an envelope from Manufacturer's Hanover. I opened it as carefully as if it were a letterbomb.

"Dear Mr. Melson:

Congratulations: You have been chosen as a candidate for our corporate training program at an annual starting salary of $28,000. Please notify us by August 31st of your intentions as classes begin September 14th.

Sincerely,
Personnel Department"

There are tear stains on that letter that are clearly visible even on photocopies.

I hit the floor. I hit the ceiling. I ricocheted off walls and broke things. I was pretty happy.

My brilliant, sappy, patriotic speech had worked! Twice what I was earning at ECIA! In my hometown newspaper's business briefs, my childhood schoolmates now working at John Deere or the Pack would read, "James Melson, graduate of Dubuque Senior

High School, has been appointed corporate banking officer at Manufacturers Hanover Trust, New York City.''

Eat your hearts out, rednecks!

Head to 54, Jimmy. *Brag.* Now you've got it all. Everyone will want you. Now if only I could handle the rigors of the program. "James Melson, graduate of Dubuque Senior High School, has been fired for flunking tests in Manufacturers Hanover Trust Company's corporate training program. He is presently unemployed.'' An outcome to be studiously avoided.

I got one solid week of all-night club hopping and crowing about James Melson, Banker, to anyone chic and beautiful out of my system; then one week of abstinence. Then the training program began. Eight groups of twenty-five trainees from the top ten schools in the country were to be put through ten to twelve months of what amounted to a corporate Marine boot camp.

I could still hear my guidance counselor at Dubuque Senior High: "James, your grades are not Ivy, but . . .''

Orientation took place in a conference room filled with classroom-type desks arranged in a semicircle. Despite my newly purchased Brooks Brothers suit, as I looked around the room I felt like a discard from K mart's bargain basement. Tasseled loafers, horn-rimmed glasses, button-down shirts, silk rep ties and suspenders were the obvious *couture de rigueur.* In alphabetical order, each person was called upon to stand up and introduce themselves and give their background. Thank God my name was not Adams, or Aalto.

With few exceptions, all were from Ivy schools; many already had MBAs. When I stood up timorously to confess my Iowa and St. Olaf roots, I felt like a barnyard animal at the gate among a lineup of thoroughbreds. At least no one broke out laughing.

It seemed a clubby bunch: they talked Ivy fraternities, rugby teams, prep schools. . . . I had nothing in common with any of them. They knew it and I knew it. When they were studying market reports in *Forbes, Barron's,* and *Business Week,* I had been improving my mind with *People, GQ,* and *Studflix.*

After the last trainee had sat down, Kathy Ballard, the program director, handed out a mountainous supply of books. Kathy was a crop-haired, mid-fortyish single woman with a dangerously bitter

look, perhaps the result of too many years of celibacy. At least as
far as men went. Some of us would later speculate about her personal life — whether she prowled the alleys of Greenwich Village,
decked out in leather, looking for a lesbian lover. She was rumored
to have been removed from her on-line lending responsibilities for
chewing out an important client about his male chauvinism. One
thing was certain — when she stood wardenlike at the front of the
class, she commanded respect, or at least abject fear.

"Okay, ladies and gentlemen," Kathy announced as she distributed the mountain of books, reports and periodicals, "this should
keep you busy for a while. We'll start with three months of macroeconomics and accounting, then three of business law and corporate
finance, one of international finance, a one month internship, then
two months of credit analysis. Periodically you will be given tests
which generally last three to four hours. If your average grades are
not 70 or above, we will have to let you go." Good luck, sleep
well, stay out of the discos, etc.

I began to sweat as if I were entering another summer of meat
packing hell, but with much higher stakes: my future. I realized that
my all-night carousing was over, at least for the duration of the
program. From now on, it was eating, drinking and sleeping banking.

All-nighters were frequent, and took a toll. The first casualty in
the group was Mary, a pretty New York State graduate whose banking future was wiped away with a sweep of a red pen on the accounting final. There were not even good-byes — she just disappeared; rumor said she'd had a nervous breakdown and had been
hospitalized. At any rate, it was clear to me that *I* was now at the
bottom of the heap, and would have to fight hard to maintain even
that exalted position.

Macroeconomics was the downfall of two more. One, a superstar
Harvard MBA, ex-captain of the rugby team and devastatingly
handsome, was rumored to have been handpicked by the bank's
Chairman McGillicuddy himself. His sex appeal had been no help
in interpreting complex financial statements. (But I could have
found a use for it.)

Our group was down to twenty-two, and I, with a 73 average,
was now next to last at the bottom of the class curve. The worst was

yet to come: the dreaded credit analysis segment, culminating in two breakless eight-hour tests in which manila folders containing hundreds of pages of financial statements, marketing, economic and industry reports were plopped on each desk. It was to be an analytical regurgitation of the previous ten months.

The tests began at 9 a.m. sharp. At 8:59 on the day of the second and final test, Kathy stood at the front of the room, checking her watch and looking forward to the slaughter. The thoroughbreds readied their pens and calculators. "Five, four, three, two, one, GO!"

For the next eight hours, no one paused except to change calculator batteries and check the clock. The test was completely bullshit-proof: no flowery verbiage could substitute for cold, hard, accurate numbers. The first to finish after 6 1/2 hours was Marty, an Einstein-like Jew — a misfit for banking, but brilliant enough to have invented quantum mechanics. The remainder of the class glanced up with groans of disbelief and despair. Pens instantly revved into fourth gear.

At 4:50, Kathy came back in. "Ten minutes and counting."

I was soaked with sweat. With each tick of the clock and punch of the calculator came visions of premature career death.

"Five minutes, please finish up."

The last of my brain circuitry was on the verge of shortage as Kathy pronounced the final countdown with stopwatch in hand: "Five, four, three, two, one. Stop working, please! Pass them in. Congratulations. You have just completed ten months of what will hopefully be the most grueling experience of your life." I crawled from the room with the other living dead, wondering how I would liquidate my no longer needed $800 Brooks Brothers wardrobe, $600 of which I owed on my new Visa card. We were all given a week's vacation; our grades would be announced the following week. On the first test, I'd scored an underwhelming 62, and I now needed a 78 or better to make the cut. So what could and should have been a wild and crazy week of sniffing coke with society luminaries in the ultraexclusive basement of Studio 54 and dancing till dawn with half-naked baby-oiled Adonises at Flamingo turned into a week of fearful waiting for the call from the hatchet woman telling me not to bother coming in the following Monday morning and that my personal belongings would be forwarded to my apartment.

That call never came; but on the training floor Monday morning, the mood was funereal. Kathy began to call us into her office, one by one, to receive either the Mark Cross pen set or the pink slip. My turn came, and I turned to take one last look at my comrades, like a pig going to slaughter.

"Mr. Melson," Kathy said, almost smiling, "congratulations. You made it by two points. We thought we lost you after the first test, Jim, but you made it like a real trooper."

I heard the rest very much as in a climactic Hollywood scene— soft lens, swelling violins, heavenly chorus. . . . But through the mist of clichés, I could just make out the gist: From now until my permanent placement, I'd be doing the same kind of analysis we'd done on the eight-hour test, only now for an actual deal. The officers were too overloaded with their calling schedules to deal with the grunt work; that is what us trainees were there for. We would have our titles, bonuses and expense accounts someday, but for now we should consider ourselves water boys (and girls). Chairman McGillicuddy is very much the sports enthusiast; the team spirit is very important, etc., etc. I was assigned to Sandra Rollins as my advisor. Only when she judged my analysis to be acceptable, i.e., perfect, would I be placed in one of three banking divisions, depending on my choice and available openings. Don't be discouraged if I couldn't be accommodated as I'd like; although I made it through, my grades were among the lowest in the class, and it went without saying that the top achievers would get first consideration. Meanwhile, here was the file on my first company: an energy group called ThermoElectron. Get in touch with Mr. Fairchild, Vice-President in charge of the account right away to let him know I was on the case.

They could have given me Duane's Villa de Coiffure in Dubuque at that point for all I cared. I left Kathy's office, gave the thumbs up to everyone and got an all-Ivy cheer. As each went in in turn, we all waited to applaud, or console. Two of them, however, never did come out. No, they hadn't jumped out the window. Kathy, it seemed, had ushered them out her office's back door to avert an unseemly display of emotion in front of the class. But was it to spare *them* embarrassment, or to avoid demoralizing *us*? Is this what corporate banking was all about? Sweep any unpleasantness under the rug? Go Team Go—but when the tight end breaks a leg, whisk him away discreetly and dispose of the remains?

I lugged the financials home that evening, wondering just what a ThermoElectron was. I could barely screw in a light bulb straight; how in Einstein's name was I going to analyze the viability of a new source of alternative energy? Why couldn't they have given me a fashion account, or better yet, something in entertainment or advertising?

I'd spent the afternoon in the bank's library with my nose buried in global market reports. It was the peak of the Middle East oil embargo, and every alternative idea from hydropower to manure was being, so to speak, floated. But start-up capital costs for such projects were tremendous, so the payoffs, if any, were speculative and long-term. In short, the deals were at best extremely risky, but the rewards could be enormous, both to the bank and to the account officer's career.

I called Mr. Fairchild early the following day.

"Okay, Jimmy, my boy, deliver for me. If I get this deal through committee, they'll believe any piece of crap I put in front of them. If you have any trouble with the numbers, round up. We want to paint a real positive picture here. You do a good job and you won't be forgotten."

What Fairchild neglected to say was that if the deal blew up, I wouldn't be forgotten either; it would be my ass for screwing up. On the one hand I had to make the numbers look good; on the other hand I knew Sandra would be checking and double-checking every single spread, cash flow and projection for the minutest of errors.

After a week of number crunching and speculative guesswork, I presented Sandra with a twenty-five-page, typed and bound analysis. Sandra was 24 years old, and pregnant. She'd been taken "off the line," ostensibly for "health reasons." The fact was, in the jock-oriented culture of MHTCo's senior management, the idea of a pregnant account officer dealing with clients was as unthinkable as the election of a black mayor in Dubuque. The only reason women were hired as account officers in the first place was pressure from the Women's movement beginning in the early 1970s.

It seemed clear to me that women like Sandra and Kathy, under-standably if unjustifiably, resented the younger men they knew would eventually overtake them, and used their positions both puni-tively and strategically, to make the men look bad and themselves good to senior management, and thus prove their own worthiness for advancement.

In other words, what Sandra did to my analysis couldn't possibly have been due to any sloppiness or incompetence on my part.

The first draft came back obliterated by her red pen. "Mr. Melson, you seemed to have missed some crucial points in your analysis. I would go so far as to suggest you shred this and start anew." The cold-hearted bitch was not going to make it easy for me.

I made endless corrections. She made endless critiques. This bat-tle of the sexes, and colors (red ink versus black) raged on for a month, by the end of which all trainees had been placed in their permanent assignments except myself. Kathy called me into her office.

"James, Sandra tells me you're having serious difficulties with your analysis. We've given you a number of shots at it and I must tell you that if your next one isn't successful we will have to let you go. You must realize here and now that test runs do not exist in the real world. If you can't assess a company's strong and weak points the first run through, and present your results clearly and convinc-ingly, you have no value to this bank. I want to see this on my desk Monday morning at nine in flawless form. I will be reviewing it this time personally." (Sandra had gone into labor. Well, she'd sure made *me* go into labor.)

So it seemed my whole *year* of labor — labor? toil, anguish, tor-ture — might leave me right where I started: unemployment. Or per-haps MHT *would* keep me — as a teller, or processing applications for K mart credit cards. My father may have bequeathed me balls and guts, but alas, he left out the brains.

I burned enough midnight oil the next few nights to constitute an alternative energy source in itself. I decided Sandra's vague criti-cisms *were* simply an expression of career frustration, and went back to my own initial ideas. Maybe Kathy would see ThermoElec-tron my way.

Monday morning I put the analysis on Kathy's desk and shrank back to my cubicle to await the verdict and death sentence. For three days and three nights the sword of Damocles or Sophocles or whoever he was dangled over my head. Finally I was summoned into Kathy's office.

"Well, James, you have once again astonished us with your comeback. The revisions you've made are excellent. You're in. And, you're very lucky to be the last to be placed; an excellent position in our Wall Street department has just opened up." I was to report to Conrad De Luca, the officer in charge, Monday morning. Wall Street, my God, my father will be bursting with pride.

I was up at six Monday to have plenty of time to primp and preen. Was the Wall Street dress code different from uptown? Suspenders and French cuffs, perhaps? Hair parted in the middle? Inconspicuous earring? Bone through the lip? Who knew? Wall Street was an exotic jungle. I did, however, know this by this point in my life: presentation was half the battle. It's a law of God. Or at least Mammon.

My trip to work, formerly a six-block walk, now involved a journey on the Subway from Hell, the Lexington Avenue line – celebrated in song and story for its 100 percent dependable mechanical breakdowns; the intimacy it afforded with one's fellow New Yorkers – and their many intriguing smells; the tropical heat, summer *and* winter, which, with the crowding, gave the city a Black Hole of Calcutta it could call its own; and the *minor* delays for removing the occasional body from the tracks – all part of that glorious pageant of accident, murder and suicide that is daily life in underground New York.

Next to the Wall Street exit, 140-year-old Trinity Church still stood fast against the ever-encroaching office towers, but wore a thick black veil of soot as though mourning Wall Street's greed. One of those towers was my destination, 40 Wall Street, a vast, brown steeple a few steps from the Stock Exchange. The street – or rather, The Street – gave little relief from the subway: narrow, hemmed in with giant buildings, jammed with pedestrians, taxis, limos, bike messengers, newspaper hawkers, all jabbering, shouting, blowing whistles, blaring horns – and it was all part of a great mill that it drove and that drove it, and that produced only one thing: money.

The MHT offices had their own elevator that opened directly onto "the floor," a cooly lit room with four rows of Chippendale-style desks, each with an emerald green glass desk lamp. The Vice President team leaders sat at the far end with their backs toward the Wall Street windows and their faces looking inward over their inferiors, like schoolteachers over their class. I was thrown immediately into the credit department, a crowded laundry-room-like area adjacent to "the floor," and given a small metal desk. Along with three others from recent training cycles, I was to have the shitwork dumped on me by the account officers. Only upon proving ourselves to the officer in charge, and personnel turnover permitting, would we be granted a desk on "the floor." Meanwhile, from here at the very bottom, we got to know the hierarchy.

At the top was Stewart Longwell, a white-haired Harvard man with horn-rimmed glasses, who rarely emerged from his corner office other than for two-hour lunches at 21 or the Union League Club. But while his Wall Street career was rooted in—indeed, almost an extension of—his old boy network of familial and collegiate athletic relationships, Longwell was now money caterer to the Boeskys, the Milkens and Wassersteins—the *arrivistes* who were rising to prominence—and notoriety—at Goldman Sachs, Drexel, Burnham, Lambert and Lehman Brothers et al. Longwell and I never met, despite the fact that he whizzed right by my desk daily, usually huffing and puffing like a pressure cooker ready to explode. His blood pressure must have been higher than the Dow-Jones average. After one of his "appointments," however, he'd return even more red-faced but slower paced, usually badmouthing the Jewish associates he had just been shmoozing for deals over a double martini lunch.

Longwell's secretary was fat Susannah Dumbrowski. Susannah, I soon found out, was known as "the tattler." She was Longwell's personal confidante; if anything or anyone got out of line on the floor, Longwell would know. Susannah lorded her power over the office staff and knew she could tell anyone to "eat shit and die" and get away with it. Whenever Longwell wanted someone from the floor, he would yell, "Susannah, get (so-and-so) in here!" and Susannah would trot off, her fat cheeks (both pairs) jiggling.

Under Longwell was the officer in charge, Conrad De Luca. The name Conrad didn't fit him; it should have been Harry, Frank or Vinny. He was a lower-middle-class Italian kid from Long Island. Sort of an East-Coast version of my father—a man with brains, drive and determination, but rough-edged and lacking the sophistication you might expect in a Wall Street banker. Corporate bankers wore blue or charcoal grey pinstripe suits, silk rep ties, and black tassel Brooks Brothers loafers. Conrad looked more like the traders or operations guys: brown suits, Countess Mara ties and Florsheim shoes. Conrad was truly a Wall Street redneck.

"Eh, Melson," his deep voice boomed. "C'mon in, relax." I knew instantly that I had a problem. His machismo intimidated me, just as my father's had intimidated me as a child. Would he sense that I was gay? Do straight men have "the sixth sense"? How deep could I lower my voice? How soon could I acquire a macho swagger?

How soon before I lost my job?

Longwell and De Luca—the old-guard WASP and the Long Island wop—made for an odd couple of leaders. They barely even communicated—but old Longwell knew what he was doing: De Luca was a rah, rah, go-team-go type of manager, and his humbler origins made him all the more bottom-line conscious and achievement-oriented. Longwell therefore could lunch and shmooze at his leisure, knowing De Luca would give him a winning year to report to the Board of Directors uptown.

The Longwell mentality flowed downwards, to the account officers; and those at the very bottom of the heap suffered for it. We were the ones who worked till eight or nine to produce the analyses to be presented to senior management uptown—while the account officers entertained clients at the U.S. Open, the Westchester Classic, and black-tie charity events.

The entire credit department staff attended bi-weekly meetings, chaired by Conrad. We gathered around an enormous leather-topped table in the imposing conference room and, one by one, presented our analyses and were then grilled by Conrad or the account officer.

My team leader, Andy Bello, had assigned me Sutro and Company, a lower-tier California brokerage firm for which he was proposing to establish a ten-million-dollar secured line of credit. Andy, a Vice President, was all of 28, and short. This young Napoleon ruled his team almost literally: he would approach my desk daily and prod me on Sutro while slapping his palm menacingly with a ruler. Finally one day he said, "Come on, Jim, I need the analysis. If we don't have quick turnaround time, Citibank's gonna get 'em. They've got a huge inventory on the books and not much capital. De Luca knows you're on it and is not all that thrilled about you. He thinks you're not of his ilk. You better kick ass to correct this impression." My initial fears seemed confirmed: De Luca *did* have the sixth sense. Well, "out" or not, I had to go *all* out preparing for Thursday morning's meeting.

Conrad began it with a pep talk to the account officers, then went on for a while about chief economist Irwin Kellner's outlook for the week, rising interest rates, plummeting collateral, preserving our clients' capital bases, and other such high drama.

"Okay, now that that's out of the way, let's hear what you flunkies got for us. You first, Melson."

Drawing on my vast public speaking experience — my performance as Dr. Graziano at Dubuque Senior High — I swallowed hard, then delivered a disgracefully meek monologue. Andy sat stunned. Then Conrad tore into me.

"Melson, you say this company's great. I think it stinks. You've completely missed the unfunded pension fund as an off-balance-sheet liability. Check the goddamn footnotes." Everyone looked down awkwardly and fidgeted while I turned beet red. "Next time, do your fucking homework."

As the meeting ended I tucked my tail between my legs and slunk back to my desk. So much for an officer title, Jimmy. You've blown it on your first try. You should have taken Andy's exhortations more to heart instead of discoing till dawn at The Saint. Why hadn't I realized completing the training program was only the beginning of the battle?

On the bright side, summer invitations to Fire Island and the Hamptons were pouring in. The Hamptons decorators wanted me as an ornament for their pastel social brunches, and the Fire Island muscle studs wanted me as their all-night disco mate and early morning sex partner. Well, I couldn't accept one group and offend the other, could I? Of course not. It had to be both.

And it *was* both, according to my mood. Each satisfied an appetite: The Hamptons, my appetite for *luxe*, and Fire Island, for sex. But both were only temporary escapes from my problems at work. And both required a Monday morning recovery: either from too much booze (the Hamptons) or too many drugs (Fire Island).

Nor did my perhaps biggest appetite — my vanity, my need to be admired — go unattended. My after-work iron pumping at the Chelsea gym continued to add to my muscle definition, and that drew the looks my ego craved. I had it all back again. And this time with substance — banking (or so I told myself). But, something was missing. There was no one to share it with. I longed for the romance of a Bud, the sexual appurtenances of a Scott, and the friendship and humor of a Keith. And in my search for a Bud or Scott or Keith I left a trail, a carnage of sexual conquests, and was in turn trailed by such epithets as whore, tramp, and size queen — based half in jealousy, half in reality.

For the sake of my reputation, (or what was left of it), I decided to stick to the Hamptons whose far more refined, indeed staid, atmosphere better befitted a banker's lifestyle than Fire Island's wildly exciting but devastatingly unhealthy weekends. I kept reminding myself that the Fire Island days should have died with my late 'seventies departure from New York to sanity. Those were the years I had to get it out of my system; and I did . . . or so I thought. But now I found that the interim years of sexual deprivation had only fed my hunger. What had I missed? My perfect match, perhaps? I still wanted to find him, more desperately than ever.

One of my first Hamptons invitations was to a party at Joe and Wally's, a handsome mid-fortyish duo I met at another party thrown by a well-known New York caterer. They were two very successful businessmen. The two ex-studs had weathered the years together and aged comfortably into a life of affluence and cocktail parties. Their invitations were among the most coveted of the Hamptons gay crowd. I could see why the moment I arrived at their house — or rather, estate. It was a sprawling, French-style country manse bordering East Hampton's Maidstone Club, Long Island's most elite country club. A long driveway led to a double-winged, mansard-roofed house with massive chimneys, carved double French doors, a swimming pool and a jacuzzi, all surrounded by several acres of flawlessly manicured grounds ensuring absolute privacy.

Wally was the Pearl Mesta of the two, chattering and gossiping at eighty miles an hour. Joe, on the other hand, was more out of the John Wayne mold: laconic, content to stand aside and watch Wally flit about, delivering his kiss-kiss, "we'll lunch" greetings and gallivanting from group to group to make sure he didn't miss one ounce of party gossip. Though, in private asides, Joe could trash with the best of them.

"Look at that decorator queen over there sipping her cocktail with Wally like she's drinking hot tea. She pals it up with the old matrons out here and shmoozes them into redecorating their houses annually with dime store junk at markups of a hundred percent or more so she can finance her stable of young fairies around her pool. Look at Wally making a fool of himself. When he's in a crowd like this he becomes one of the girls. Bunch of sissy prima donnas. Stay away from them, they're nothing but cheap gay trash."

I instantly identified with Joe. He was like a gay version of my father. I could be open with him. I shared his interest in Americana, such as the antique duck decoys which lined the bookshelves of his walnut-paneled den. We became friends. We'd sit for hours in front of his fireplace at night or at his poolside during the day, talking about business, the economy, his world travels, and—especially important to me—his dual identity as a gay corporate executive. He had achieved astounding success despite what was, in the man's world of big business, a severe social handicap: though as masculine as anyone could want, he didn't have a wife. How did he handle cocktail parties and dinners with business associates and their spouses? He explained that, first, his area was operations rather than sales; therefore, client exposure was minimal. Secondly, whenever called upon for any business/pleasure "do," he pleaded "too much work," and delegated the social duties to some always-eager subordinate.

Joe and Wally had lived for years as the Adonis and Donatello of New York. Whereas Wally had graduated gracefully from the more sexual stage of life to the more social, Joe was having difficulty making the transition. Despite his disparagement of the decorators' "keeping" boys, Joe periodically drove his Jaguar down to the gay beach at night where cars would line up with lights turned off and wait as young entrepreneurs paraded by, offering their stuffed baskets in exchange for stuffed pockets. Joe secretly did his thing and returned home. But I knew that these brief, dark, faceless encounters did not satisfy Joe's passion for youth, which if anything grew as his own youth receded. Not that he ever so much as broached such an encounter with me; he knew he'd be risking the loss of my companionship. Instead, ours grew more and more into a father-son relationship.

And a rewarding one, even beyond the companionship. A guest suite overlooking the pool became mine for the asking. Soon after, a brand new Jeep CJ-7 was purchased for my use, as neither Joe nor Wally considered it appropriate for me to be seen driving the Jaguar or the Eldorado; too much like the decorators' "kept" boys. Not that Joe didn't enjoy showing me off in public, *especially* to the decorator cocktail crowd he so intensely loathed. But whenever he introduced me, he always emphasized my Wall Street position so as to imply my interest in him was other than monetary. He took pleasure in the queeny, gossipy speculation about our "carnal" relationship. Thus, the benefits were mutual: Joe could maintain his image as a Hamptons stud, and I could enjoy all the material advantages of the son of a Fortune 500 chieftain.

But I had to watch it. As much as material possessions and status counted among the Hamptons crowd, on Fire Island it was different. There it was a live-for-the-moment, muscle-pumping, sex, drugs, and rock and roll crowd. And it was my Fire Island reputation I wanted to preserve — and protect from jealousy and gossip about Joe and me — for it was this group that comprised the eligible stable for choosing a long-term mate. The frail young WASPs clothed in blue blazers with bogus family crests, signet rings, and monogrammed everything, offered nothing, sexually. They didn't have it and wouldn't know how to use it if they did. But there again, it was a delicate balancing act: As I had learned during my first stay in New York, too much exposure in any one locale tended to evaporate one's mystique — a new face could quickly turn into a has-been;

so I showed my face (and body) at the Pines just often enough not to be forgotten.

At one of Joe and Wally's decorator soirees, among the paunch and pastel crowd downing their cocktails at a competitive pace, I ran into Chad Wilson. Chad was from Farmerville, Louisiana, and the son of a funeral home owner; yet he had somehow transformed himself into an irresistible blend of Southern hillbilly and thoroughly Manhattan, thoroughly worldly cafe-society social maven, whose black humor, outrageous send-ups of the old-guard Southern mentality, and perfect impersonation of Aretha Franklin invariably sent his "audiences" reeling in gut-wrenching laughter. He had shmoozed his way into a job with the couturier house of Mollie Parnis, and from that base had gone on to establish an impressive array of social contacts.

Chad told me his roommate André was moving to San Francisco, and asked if I was interested in moving in. He lived at none other than "Four out of Five" — 405 East 58th, the same building as — in fact just down the hall from — Jon Murray, the sadomasochistic supermodel who had once thrown me out for being an S&M party pooper.

Chad seemed like perfect roommate material: worldly, well connected, with flawless taste and a superb sense of humor. And he was evidently elated at the prospect of adding me to his collection of prized *objets*, art and antiques.

I gave Spencer the news. His reaction, understandably, was poorly concealed regret; he knew my move meant that his romantic ambitions vis-à-vis *moi* would now never be realized.

Meanwhile, back at the office, I'd been expecting a Junior Officer title, specifically Assistant Treasurer, but was passed by in favor of two people from subsequent cycles: Mary Beth de Filippes, an Amy Vanderbilt-like deb from Greenwich, and orange-haired Seymour Klein, the quintessential Jewish geek.

Bitter about being held back, I hit the headhunters. What I really wanted — really, *really* wanted — was to switch to investment banking; the seven-figure salaries and Hamptons houses were the envy of every lowly commercial banker. I prepared my résumé, inflated it to Hindenburg proportions, and mailed it out. Soon after, my secretary said a Joe Franklin was on the line.

"Jim, this is really Peter Sedgewick; I don't like to use my real name. Headhunting, as I'm sure you know, is a clandestine operation. We've got a position you might be interested in just down the street at Credit Suisse. You'd be responsible for starting up an investment banking department. I think it could be a real coup. Credit Suisse has huge depository reserves at low rates while money center banks are supporting their loans by buying money through the Fed. Offer a rate of anything less than seventy-five basis points and you'll have every CFO clamoring to get your money."

God, I said, how I'd love to steal business away from Conrad De Luca.

I met with Jeffrey Westcott, a yupped-out VP with tassel loafers, suspenders, power tie, slicked-back hair and Cartier tank watch — the antithesis of De Luca. It was obvious at first glance he was king of the shmoozers. We hit it off immediately and I felt that I had the job sewn up. Within a week, a formal offer arrived in the mail:

"Congratulations. Credit Suisse is pleased to offer you the position of Assistant Treasurer, Investment Banking, at a starting salary of $40,000."

Yeehaw! Kiss off, De Luca! Eat shit, Longwell! In about so many words, I gleefully composed my letter of resignation.

My glee was very soon overshadowed. After all-night partying at The Saint, the next afternoon I noticed a strange rash covered with little pus-filled blisters on my left leg. What kind of herpetic virus could I have contracted? It seemed to be spreading by the minute. I called my doctor for an appointment.

Dr. Jasper told me I had a case of the shingles and that there was really nothing he could do. By this point the blisters had completely engulfed my calf, and were giving me excruciating pain, not to mention soaking my pant leg with drainage. What does this mean? I asked. Is it sexually transmitted? Is it contagious? None of the doctor's answers suggested it was a sign of a severely weakened immune system. Unbeknownst to either of us, it was the first symptom of my ultimate reckoning.

Chapter 10

The Not-So-Innocents Abroad

How much a dunce that has been sent to roam excels a dunce
that has been kept at home.

— William Cowper

That September, 1983, I decided it was time I visited Europe at
long last.

I had recently met David Felker, a fellow muscle pumper at the
gym. David had attended the Johns Hopkins School of International
Politics in Bologna, Italy, and wanted to make a return trip to renew
his friendships there. Talking in the sauna, I told him of my own
liking for Italians — how I found them so sleek and sophisticated and
at the same time sensuous and darkly sexy.

With us was Julio Morales. The son of a nouveau riche Mexican
immigrant, Julio was a graduate of the State University of New
York and a would-be businessman. But unlike me, he hadn't had
the luck of meeting a George Harris to open doors for him; so he
spent his days endlessly mailing out résumés and working out his
frustrations at the gym, which had at least yielded him an admirable
physique, of which a faultless washboard stomach was the chief attraction. Our conversation aroused his interest. Julio spoke French
and had twice been to Paris. With David fluent in Italian and me
nearly able to get by in German, we seemed the linguistically perfect
team for "doing Europe."

Within days we had booked our flight on Icelandic Air, the
cheapest overseas fare available. The catch: a two-hour layover in
Reykjavik and destination of Luxembourg. Well, when else would I
ever visit Iceland or Luxembourg?

Europe had always seemed as remote as the moon — and my expectations were as high. It would be the next and crowning stage, after New York, in my education. I had graduated from bib overalls to Brooks Brothers; now for my doctorate: Armani and Versace. After all, if you didn't own a hot leather jacket purchased in Milan or Florence, you were a bumpkin.

Over an appropriate three-stage meal — French wine and pâté de foie gras at Le Relais, pasta and chianti at Trattoria da Alfredo and dark German beers at the Hofbrau House — David, Julio and I planned our itinerary: We would rent a car and drive to Paris, spend three days, proceed east and south through Germany and Switzerland, then down into Italy, to Florence, Portofino and Rome. David would remain in Bologna and Julio and I would drive back to Luxembourg for our return flight.

It was a lot for two weeks, but I insisted on no less. If I'd had my way, London would have been thrown in too, but David brought me back to my senses: "Jimmy, if you want to do all of Europe in two weeks the only memories you'll have of it will be from a car window."

Oh, I wanted some indoor memories, all right, just not that sort. And as the evening and the drinking went on, the talk turned to the sexier part of the itinerary: Julio's fantasies about Jean Pierres and Michels, mine about Vittorios and Paolos, and David — David just blushed and giggled like a little schoolgirl. Julio and I tried to help him out by suggesting that maybe his fantasy was to be licked in the face by a St. Bernard in the Alps.

We stumbled out of the Hofbrau House in the wee hours like three drunken collegiates celebrating a winning game. David grabbed a cab home to the Upper East Side. Julio lived in Hoboken, New Jersey. He asked if I'd like to come and see the Manhattan skyline from the poor folks' side of the river, his eyes twinkling to suggest more than a pretty night view. "Sounds like the perfect opportunity to start a journal of our trip," I said. "Might even prove to be the highlight." We took the subway to Penn Station to catch the Path train under the Hudson.

The Path train at 2 a.m. reminded me of my first solo subway ride to the Loop in downtown Chicago. Pale ghostly figures with vacant eyes, some drinking out of paper bags, others snorting coke, others babbling or arguing with invisible companions — and everywhere the smells of every conceivable bodily discharge. Such a perfect romantic prelude. The reader may wish to note for future reference that the Path train to New Jersey is the most effective anti-aphrodisiac yet discovered. I can't be exact, but I'd say my libido got off at Christopher Street.

Hoboken itself was something of a relief: a mixed community with a solid base of Italians — the sort I'd come to know from the operations departments on Wall Street — and an overlay of new-comers: artists, yuppies, gentrifiers — refugees from Manhattan.

Though Julio fell somewhere in the latter category, the apartment he shared on the second floor of a large unrenovated brownstone was a model of tackiness; orange shag carpeting, waterbed . . . lava lamp! One look and I knew he was not long-term relationship material. Nevertheless, I was stuck for the night, drunk in Hoboken (a solo trip back to Manhattan on the Path was out of the question). Besides, the lure of Julio's prizewinning abdomen was not to be passed up.

Like a real trooper, I'd come through the train ride *and* the tacky decor, and was still, so to speak, standing; battle-hardened. The next test of the, uh, firmness of my resolve was the waterbed. I'd never tried one; and in my inexperience, inebriation, and eagerness I made a swan dive onto it, creating a tidal wave that washed poor Julio clear overboard. The embarrassment rendered my member as squishy as the mattress. But Julio climbed back on board, and once I started running my hands up and down his rippling tummy, my tumescence recovered.

Up to this point I had not seen Julio totally naked. David and I took our saunas in the nude, but Julio, exasperatingly, always wore a towel. Now, at this moment of truth, I found out why. This poor, unfortunate man was afflicted with penile anorexia. The organ in question was so thin, so pencil-like, I feared it might break off in my hand with the first couple of strokes. For the third time in an hour, my willie wilted with disappointment.

Not so Julio. Well, then, let him have his way with me. I lay there passively as he slid his wire up and down my leg like a chihuahua in heat. Thankfully, at least he finished his business quickly. Less thankfully, despite what I thought was my obvious lack of enthusiasm, Julio's eyes indicated hopes for more than a one-night roll in the hay.

Julio's tackiness, joblessness and dicklessness, and David's shy little-girlishness had dashed my hopes for a relationship with one of the two to complete my romantic European holiday. There was no bowing out now; our tickets were noncancelable, nonrefundable and nonchangeable. But at the very least I had to find a way to fend off their advances and leave myself free to forage for my own. The next day, I asked my roommate Chad for advice.

"Jimmy, give Julio your 'Sorry, I don't smoke' line when he offers it to you, and buy David a *Playgirl* magazine. This is *your* time in Europe. It's your vacation. You've worked your butt off the past year and you deserve the best. Honey, if you hadn't hooked up with those two losers, with that blond mop on your head you'd be given carte blanche with the crème de la crème of every hot-blooded European stud you set your eyes on. All you'd have to do is step into La Coupole alone and you'd be deluged with invites to every chateau, villa and yacht from the Loire to the Tiber. Take advantage of their splitting the room costs and their language abilities, then take off on your own. Just beware of the Eurotrash. They'll try to impress you with their aristocratic lineages and hand-me-down titles and you'll end up in bed the next morning lucky if you have your underwear left."

Preposterous and fantastic though the picture of glamour he painted was, it was my kind of fantasy, and just the cheering up I needed. And with any luck, David and Julio would strike up a romance between themselves, and I could run around on my own, free of any guilt.

Two weeks later we landed in Iceland, where, though it was October, we were met with bitter cold, and of course, ice. We rushed into the terminal, where the first people we saw were three pasty-faced Icelandic hillbillies enjoying their favorite pastime — hanging out at the airport and gawking at the foreigners. Life in Iceland must be exciting, I thought. Much like working at the Pack in Dubuque.

Julio, though jobless, was well financed by his father, and he immediately set about impressing David and me with his spending, buying Icelandic sweaters and expensive hiking boots at the airport store without batting an eye. Well, more power to him. I was saving every penny for that leather jacket in Florence or Milan.

We took off again for Luxembourg. I couldn't wait to see the view of lofty castle turrets that would greet us on our approach. As we began our descent I searched in vain for my Disneyland towers. Below was nothing more than Iowa-like agriland. Where were the Schloss-Neuschwansteins I'd seen photos of in my architectural history class at St. Olaf? This was not what I had expected of my first glimpse of Europe.

Upon touchdown I was awestruck at finally being in Europe, *and* struck by how mundane everything looked. If I didn't know better I would have sworn we'd landed in Omaha or Des Moines. Had I spent my life savings on an extravagant overseas jaunt in the company of two nonentities for *this*, when a trip home to Dubuque would have cost one-tenth as much? Well, I thought, already figuring out how to salvage what I could, at least I could return home the world-wise traveler, able to cast well-informed pearls before the less well-traveled swine, able to hold my own among the international set — no longer the Iowa ignoramus afraid to open his mouth for fear of sticking his foot in it.

Upon "deplaning" I posed momentarily at the top of the stairs like Brigitte Bardot arriving at the Cannes Festival gazing towards the crowd beyond the gate and awaiting an explosion of flash bulbs from an army of paparazzi. How quickly I could shift from disappointment to daydream . . .

While David dealt with the baggage claim, I insisted Julio accompany me to the car rental hoping he could book a Mercedes or BMW touring car before budget-conscious David could veto our extravagance. I needn't have worried. I had made my currency exchange well in advance, getting seven French francs to the dollar; but, despite my bank training in international finance, I had ignored the weekly economic reports, and had no idea of the franc's real value. I thought 7,000 francs would carry me through Europe in ultra-luxury. I was floored when the concierge at the car rental agency quoted us a weekly rate of 6,800 francs for a basic 260D. Which did I want, a fleeting two-week memory of Europe from a Mercedes, or Europe in a Ford Fairlane *and* a chic leather jacket — a status symbol I could take home and show off to all the boys at The

Saint? No contest. Take the status home. I'd had my BMW; my car-obsessed days were supposedly over. Anyway, David definitely *would* have nixed the idea. From what I had gathered, during his student days in Bologna he'd supported himself by stomping grapes for wine, peasant-style. He obviously had different ideas about how to do Europe. But although I conceded on the car issue, I was damned if I was going to survive in Italy on pizza slices and cheap wine at roadside tavernas. I wanted to see and be seen in the best of Europe's restaurants and discotheques. How was I going to end up on a yacht on the Riviera with Ponti and his stable of starlets by wandering around the Uffizi with a bunch of camera-laden tourists? Although not overly endowed with brainmatter, by now I had learned that presentation *wasn't* everything; you also needed entrée, and gaining entrée depended on being in the right place at the right time with the right people.

The countryside between Luxembourg and Paris looked little different than that between Dubuque and Des Moines. Where were the stone fences, the quaint half-timbered, thatched-roof houses I had seen in *Travel and Leisure?* Knowing Julio was no stranger to France, I punished him with nonstop criticism for not finding a more scenic route. And such was my touchiness that I imagined his every conversation with a gas station attendant to be a torrent of scorn aimed at me.

Compounding my crankiness was the prospect of the sleeping arrangements in our budget accommodations, where we would toss a coin for the single bed and two would have to share the double. The thought of ending up with girlish David or penis-deficient Julio rubbing against me almost made me yearn for the wide open spaces of the American Midwest.

We arrived in the City of Light around midnight to be confronted with "No Vacancy" signs everywhere. Julio had assured us that advance reservations were not necessary. My anger was now near tantrum level. Finally, after driving around in endless circles, a sputtering red neon light (much like my state of mind) said "Vacancy." Under the light hung a rusted tin sign—"Hotel Julienne." Ah, an affiliate of the seedy Julien Hotel in downtown Dubuque.

We rang the buzzer seventeen or eighteen times until a short, scruffy, baggy-eyed innkeeper finally appeared in dirty robe and holey slippers. As we made our way to the dilapidated front desk, Julio apologized for waking him at such a late hour, but without much effect. Obviously irritated at being awakened and even more irritated that we were Americans, he demanded cash up front—no credit cards, no traveler's checks. Exhausted, we made our way up the creaky flights to our room.

I had worried for nothing whether I would get the single bed: there was none; only one double. I immediately volunteered to take the floor, in exchange for the room's sole pillow. Better yet, the red neon sign was right outside our window (this seemed to be my fate), and no corner of the room escaped its garish glow. And the room smelled. No wonder there were vacancies. No doubt there were worse places to stay in Paris—such as a bench in a Metro station, or beneath a bridge. Its sole claim to class was that, unlike the Julien-Dubuque, there were no sex holes in the walls.

The next day was not much better. Our first stop was to be the Eiffel Tower. We found it covered girder to girder with some sort of netting. Somehow I didn't remember this part of the design from my architectural history class at St. Olaf. Near the entrance was a sign, "Danger, fermé pour renovations." After the previous day's misery, I hoped my first day in Paris would be as wondrous as a child's in Disneyland. So far it was as satisfying as accompanying Dad through the livestock exhibits at the Dubuque County Fair. Perhaps I was paying some sort of obligatory dues for the romp through Europe's discos and the sex, drugs, and rock and roll still to come.

Disappointed, we walked to the Champs-Élysées and planted ourselves at a sidewalk café with a view to viewing the wealthy, ultrachic French promenading by in their new Armanis and Diors. But what odd French these were; they almost all looked and spoke exactly like people from Chicago, Denver, Dusseldorf, Melbourne, Osaka—and, for that matter, Dubuque, Iowa. Well, if the French wanted to masquerade as Germans and Japanese and Americans, then I would pretend to be French. As they walked by gawking at us, I looked down my nose at them all in my most supercilious, *mangez la merde* fashion.

Up to this point, the French had kept a perfect record: Not one had acknowledged any knowledge of English—indeed, they all seemed to revel in my linguistic frustration. The waiter here did not let us down. I asked him for help in interpreting the menu: "Je regret, monsieur, mais . . ." Well, then, I knew it couldn't hurt his feelings if, as he handed us the bill, I remarked that he looked like a fey, bitchy little queen. Imagine my surprise, then, when he spit at my feet and called me "American pig." Julio and David could not have been more amused. Charmed, and sorry to have to leave our French hosts, we made our way back to the hotel to prepare to continue on our way to Germany, Switzerland and Italy.

Outside Kitzbuhl, in the middle of the Alps, my stomach began to rumble.

"Oh, my God, not the Turkish trots."

Julio, the self-appointed driver, had to stop every few miles so I could let loose, usually behind a tree or rock outcropping.

Then we entered the Simplon, the longest tunnel in the world, connecting Switzerland and Italy. There is simply no stopping in the Simplon.

"Oh, my God." Somewhere between Switzerland and Italy, in the bowels of the Alps, I was compelled to let loose. Grade 2 revisited: the poop man rides again. Gagging and groans of disgust from Julio and David.

"Why couldn't you have held it?"

"I'm afraid it's hereditary; no holding power."

David brought out a small aerosol can of deodorizer and sprayed the car as Julio gritted his teeth and floored the pedal to ninety.

We emerged to find strikingly different scenery. The pristine, Heidi-like chalets and flawless road signage of Switzerland were replaced by falling stucco and tile-roofed houses and pothole-filled roads. We continued our drive south and reached Florence, where we went about exploring the arts, climbing to the top of the Duomo, and most important, navigating the back streets in search of the Crisco disco where I had high hopes of finding my Donatello.

Finally, after walking in circles for hours, about two blocks from the Via Calzaivoli we heard the unmistakable gay disco beat. Our feet followed our ears down a dark alley, passing by swarthy, thick-lipped Italians right out of *L'uomo*, *Vogue*, or *Blueboy* for that matter. "I think we're heading in the right direction," I shrewdly deduced.

Suddenly, there it was — the neon sign of the Crisco Club. Bingo, at long last. An intimidating, unshaven doorman demanded to see our IDs. When he saw our New York licenses he immediately yelled to his friend, "New York, New York, Village Piple, Paolo, the Village Piple."

Paolo, a very young employee, went swirling into the DJ booth and within seconds a most distasteful "Macho, Macho Man" was blaring over the speakers. Embarrassed at being identified with the stereotype Christopher Street fags, I was about to make an about-face when David pointed out a stunning creature with a classical aquiline nose and droopy Stallone-like eyes, decked out in Versace. He approached and David made the introductions. Drooling over this Italian masterpiece named Giancarlo, I suddenly loathed David and his knowledge of the language. Giancarlo, alas, spoke no English. How could I possibly make any romantic overtures to anyone without verbal communication? It was obvious from the lively conversation between David and Giancarlo that David had struck gold. That left me with Julio for the rest of the evening, who was no doubt already calculating that with David preoccupied, he and I would head back to the room for a night of passionate, abandoned *amore*. *Questa è bella*! (That's a good one!)

Seething over David's coup, Julio and I headed in uncomfortable silence back to our pensione. How am I going to tactfully fend him off? Dysentery. Yes, that's the answer. Good old dysentery. Although mine had subsided since the tunnel, I insisted we make pit stops at tavernas on the way back to the room so I could credibly fake a relapse. That ought to get me out of his system. So to speak.

Worked like a charm — or should I say a purgative? — and soon I was enjoying a well-earned sleep.

About 4 a.m. a drunken David came bounding into the room. "Amore, amore, viva Italia, viva Italia, bella, bellissimo!"

Startled, Julio and I looked at each other and burst out laughing.

"Well, Julio, looks like David enjoyed pepperoni for dessert, or was it salami?"

David just gushed and giggled and said, "I'm not the type to kiss and tell, guys; you'll have to use your imagination."

Shit, Day Four gone by with nothing but misery.

The next day we wandered through the Uffizi, perusing dickless marble statues and faking artistic awe. Obviously, Michelangelo was unfamiliar with John Holmes. Finally, after persistent pestering I managed to extricate the two of them from the museum in favor of shopping on the Via Lungaro Orcini for the legendary leather jacket.

In a designer leather boutique called John F., a leather jacket screamed "buy me, buy me" (or "comprimi, comprimi"). How appropriate to have a John F. jacket for my Florence club debut at Jackie O., the most chic of the city's clubs. I had to have it, even if the $450 price meant pizza slices and hot dogs for the rest of the trip. As I signed my traveler's checks, I glanced at my companions to find David green with envy (unless he was getting dysentery too) and Julio looking hateful and not about to be outdone. Sure enough, a block away Julio darted into a place called Leonardo's and nonchalantly dropped $1,200 for the most expensive jacket in the store. David and I just looked at each other dumbstruck as Julio flounced and gloated like Zsa Zsa showing off a new Russian sable. We had to toil our tails off to scrimp and save for the trip, while Julio spent Daddykins's money as if it was tap water. Fine. We decided to turn off our attention and ignore him as much as possible. Let him pay.

Three grown men, see how they bitch . . . .

We went on to Portofino, playground of the rich and famous on the Italian Riviera. Alas, the rich and famous proved elusive. They were there — the lineup of sleek yachts moored in the harbor testified to that. I decided to take a solo walk up and down the docks with a lost-puppy-dog look in hopes that I would be invited aboard somewhere for an afternoon of champagne and caviar and hobnobbing with the glitterati. Sure that David and Julio's presence would ruin my chances, I told them I was just going out to look for postcards. Sure enough, after a half hour on the docks, David and Julio turned up.

"Find any good cards?" they smirked.

"Gentlemen," I repeated, "take it from one with experience. Being with the right people at the right time in the right place is the key to happiness." Well, I thought sadly, maybe the three vectors would converge in Rome, where, after all, all roads lead.

And where ours led us next — and fast, thanks to Julio's maniacal driving. My nerves were frazzled by time we pulled into Rome's

Anglo-American Hotel, where a cherubic desk clerk with a Dali-like mustache greeted us with much enthusiasm.

"Americano, what it like, real blond weemen? I like. Weemen here want look Marilyn Monroe, but it no work."

An Italian Quasimodo of a bellboy loaded our luggage on a cart and trudged down a worn path on the cigarette-burned, chartreuse carpeting to the elevator.

The room was actually a suite; I made sure I'd have privacy in my last days in Italy for a potential tryst with some swarthy Don Giovanni. We settled in and consulted our Bob Damron's Italy guidebook, the gay Fodor's, for the hottest night spot. Another Jackie O. seemed to be the choicest of clubs. We walked down the Spanish steps and meandered through the Piazza Navona, drooling over Italian hustlers standing around waiting for their next client.

Jackie O. was a glitzy club, seemingly home to a disappointing crowd of straights and assorted Mafiosi. The shrill eardrum-shattering music was enough to drive anyone away. A scotch on the rocks cost twelve dollars. At this point all I had left was money for the bus from JFK into New York.

On our last night, we were trudging disappointedly back to the hotel when a handsome young Italian pulled up next to us on a BMW motorcycle.

"Americano?"

"Why, yes. Italiano?" (I didn't really think he was Albanian or Taiwanese.)

With an enchanting gaze that well-nigh melted me into a puddle, he introduced himself as Alfredo. "You ride with me? I show you city on back of bike."

Talk about a deus ex machina. The thought of hugging this gorgeous Italian stud-meat as we raced around the now-vacant streets made my prick stand on end. We completed the introductions. Alfredo was a clothing designer; the sumptuous black leather jacket he was wearing was, he said, one of his designs. I looked at a fuming Julio, straddled the bike, wrapped my arms around Alfredo's midsection and bid the two "arrivederci."

Alfredo drove as if he were the lead in some Italian moto-cross. The exhilarating ride should have scared the bejesus out of me, but it was more like I'd died and gone to heaven holding onto this gorgeous creature.

Alfredo took my hand from his stomach and lowered it onto his swollen crotch, and I do mean swollen. I unzipped his leather pants and put my hand around his giant uncut Italian sausage, stroking it up and down like a piston as we raced around the Vatican. Just as we passed the Trevi fountain, Alfredo moaned as he shot a fountain of jism onto his handlebars.

I told him I should really get back to the hotel as I needed to prepare for an early morning departure to drop David in Bologna before we headed back to New York. Alfredo looked at me with his coal black pools and kissed me with his sensual Italian lips. (An Italian should always have Italian lips.) I reciprocated with a hug and one last grab of his crotch for posterity's sake. At long last, my Italian fantasy had been fulfilled.

I entered the hotel room to be greeted by the silent treatment. Va bene. That's fine. I went to sleep with a smile on my face, still smelling the lingering aroma of Alfredo's leather. At 6 a.m., after a continental breakfast of mudlike coffee and petrified croissants, we loaded the car and headed north to Bologna. When we pulled into David's Italian family's humble home, a posse of screaming bambini ran out and engulfed David's legs with little viselike grips.

Mona Giovannini, a massive woman with breasts that rested on her prodigious and prolific belly, threw her great arms around David and gave him an eye-popping squeeze. Then she herded us into the dining room where a large table was laden with mountains of pasta.

"Mangiate, mangiate." David practically did a swan dive into a bowl of linguini, as though eager to add to his spare tire and perhaps one day match Signora Giovannini.

After the gorge I suggested it was time Julio and I leave as we had to drive through the night in order to catch our midafternoon flight from Luxembourg.

Alone in the car with Julio for twenty-five hours; what a treat. We drove through the Italian countryside in solemn silence. As we ascended into the mountains, it started to snow. This was no deterrent for Julio, who swerved back and forth at high speed. Clutching my seat belt for dear life, I couldn't take it any longer.

"Goddamit, Julio, slow down or let me drive."

"Hell, no. I know what I'm doing."

"Yeah, you're trying to kill me."

When the customs agent at the Italian-Swiss border asked to see our passports, I handed mine to Julio and we were directed through. About a mile later I asked Julio for my passport back. He opened his window and tossed it out.

"Are you fucking out of your mind?" I floored the brake pedal with my foot and we swerved back and forth to a stop just inches away from the edge of a cliff. I jumped out of the car to retrieve my passport and Julio floored the gas, leaving me stranded on the cold, desolate mountain. I trudged through the snow for about a mile. Finally, headlights approached; it was Julio. I guess the bastard had second thoughts. I hopped in, slammed the door, and lunged at his neck. He punched me in the jaw.

How could I stand being in the car with this maniac for another twelve hours? I climbed into the backseat for my medicine kit, downed two valiums and went to sleep.

Unshaven, dirty and exhausted, we pulled into the airport. Without a word, I gathered my luggage, hopped out, slammed the door and headed for the check-in counter.

I arrived back in New York after a seemingly endless flight and cabbed it into the city. In the midst of fumbling with the triple lock of the apartment door, the door suddenly opened to a fat black drag queen in a caftan and transparent plastic hair bag.

"Can I help you, sir?"

Oh, God, what's Chad up to now?

Chad peered from around the corner.

"Come in, hon. How was Europe? Find any titles to marry? Oh, I got us a maid. You are just too messy to deal with. Jim, meet Bobbi; that's Bobbi with an i."

She thrust forth a limp wrist. "Charmed, I'm sure." Chad's pretentiousness seemed to have already rubbed off on her. Maybe she thought Chad was keeping me, and didn't realize I was going to be paying half her salary.

"Great, Chad. Everything I own is filthy dirty; does she do laundry?"

"Of course."

The next night there was a Winter Olympics party at Studio. I was dying to show off my new leather jacket and Missoni sweater, jet lag or no jet lag. And every hot athlete in the world would be there, dancing his sinewy heart out. I cabbed over and stooped into a crowd of sheer mayhem. A body-building show was in progress. Oh, how the dickless muscleheads enjoyed wetting the pussies of the nubile young debs. Their skimpy swimsuits were beginning to bulge — not with mutual admiration but with the money, hotel room keys and vials of coke the Muffys and Dee Dees were stuffing them with.

One of Studio's famed dancing bartenders (he was poetry in motion, stirring and shaking far beyond the call of duty) spotted me, poured me a gin and tonic and handed me four drink cards — one with his phone number on the back. "Catch me on my break and we'll go down to the basement for some toot."

When he got off at 4 a.m., he asked me to go home with him. With his moves and his packed pouch, he didn't have to beg me. We headed out the back door to a waiting limo, one of his many perks in reward for his star quality.

His Upper West Side apartment looked like a set from *American Gigolo*; everything high-tech with a bed built into a platform in Donghia greys. He stripped, exposing an awesome ass and sizeable equipment, then brought out a bottle of Dom Perignon and a vial of coke. It was party time.

He was a wild animal, and during a break from our sex I noticed blood on the sheets. My rectum had been punctured.

Two or three years before, I might not have given it a second thought. But it was 1983 now, and the only conceivable question was, what if he was positive?

Chapter 11

Nikos

It's not the men in my life that counts — it's the life in my men.

—Mae West

On New Year's Eve, Spencer held a pre-Saint dinner for eight in the Village. The group included a noted financial columnist; an ultrayuppy investment banker from Lake Forest, Illinois; his lover, a hyped-out commodities trader; Spencer and his date, an airheaded model who didn't know his ass from a hole in the ground; and myself. We met for cocktails at Spencer's, had dinner at Trattoria da Alfredo, went home for our disco naps and regrouped at The Saint at 1 a.m.

The place was elbow to elbow, and tush to tush. I had dropped a magic mushroom which was just kicking in when, looking over the bare-chested crowd, I made eye contact with a dead ringer for a young Burt Reynolds, wearing black cowboy boots and faded red 501 jeans, with a knockout face and physique, short-cropped dark brown hair and deep, dark eyes. He came up to me smiling.

"Hi, my name is Nikos. I am from Greece. I am studying at New York University. Would you like to dance?" Well, if he was studying at NYU, I guess it was all right. I nodded and followed his godlike gluteus maximi up the spiral stairs to the dance floor. This was a vast area under a mammoth dome onto which was projected a planetarium display of the night sky. With the added booster rockets of my mushroom, I felt like I had gone to homo heaven. As we stepped onto the dance floor, the crowd parted for us like the Red Sea parted for Moses.

From the swarm of half-naked men here lost in self-abandon, you wouldn't know there was such a thing as AIDS, or that the new watchword was monogamy. For many of them, the battle between compulsive sex and common sense, and the message implicit in the songs the DJ now flipped on — "Tainted Love" and "Love Kills" — were lost. But not me — not any longer. I felt that everything I had searched for in Europe and for years before had come to me in the divine shape of Nikos. My search, and its attending trail of carnage, was over. Arm in arm and drenched in sweat we paraded each other around so all could see what we had found; the pride of ownership, you might say. We made our way to the banquette to take a breather. I stared into the dark pools of Nikos's eyes and kissed his sensual Mediterranean lips. I was in love again.

I looked at my watch and was shocked to find it was nearly 6 a.m.

"Nikos, how would you like to come home with me?"

"I think I'd like that very much."

My pupils were still dilated from the hallucinogen, and as we emerged into the dawn, the light was blinding. Cabs were lined up like planes during rush hour at La Guardia. Once back at 405 East 58th we tiptoed past the dozing doorman. Inside, I flipped Vangelis on the stereo as Nikos excused himself to the bathroom. Minutes later the door opened and out he came, buck naked with a raging hard-on which took my breath away. I brought him into my bed and proceeded to lick and suck the beautiful piece of flesh for hours until he quivered and ejaculated what seemed like gallons of cum. We then took quaaludes to bring us down and curled up like spoons for the day's sleep.

"I'm scared, Nikos."

"Scared of what, Jim?"

"I'm afraid that when I wake up I won't find you sexy, or you me. I mean, these mushrooms really affect your judgment."

"Well, time will tell if either of us is disappointed. Let's just remember this night as one of the best in our lives."

Around three in the afternoon I was awakened by Nikos's hardened pole rubbing up against my rear. I was almost scared to see what I had brought home, but to my relief the creature lying next to me was as beautiful as the night before.

I was famished, and suggested we dine with Chad at the Mayfair just several blocks south. On our way out through the lobby we met Hermione Gingold coming in with her little Yorkshire terrier and with her wig on backwards. Age was taking a toll on the old gal's mind.

The restaurant catered to older, well-heeled Upper East Side homosexuals. As we were seated at our booth, Chad suddenly turned white as a ghost. "Oh, my God, it's Jon Murray." I turned to see the emaciated, balding figure that was all that remained of the once-gorgeous supermodel. "I heard that he's got the big A and is selling his glass collection at Christie's next week." Thank God our little, shall we say, tête-à-tête had not worked out. The sight of him haunted me for days.

Nikos and I were so enamored of each other that we sequestered ourselves in bed for four days of unrelenting passion. Then we went to see Nikos's place. It was a dismal five-floor walkup on Thompson Street in the Village, totally unbefitting the scion of a rich Greek he said he was. I began to wonder about that. His roommate Bill greeted me with unmistakable hostility. His interest in Nikos must have gone beyond cohabitation.

Nikos's bedroom was slightly bigger than a walk-in closet and had a homemade loft bed; Bill slept above, Nikos below. After two weeks of our alternating between Nikos's place and mine, it was obvious that Bill was tired of sharing his bedroom (as was Chad, with whom I shared a studio). It all came to a head one night when Nikos and I were going at it with such astonishing energy that the shaking of the loft bed must have measured at least 8.5 on the Richter scale. Suddenly from the loft overhead, Bill roared, "Enough is enough, this is the last straw. I can't get a wink of sleep. Either you're out or I am." The poor soul, hopelessly in love with Nikos, had finally realized that I was not just another fleeting fuck date. The next day Bill let Nikos know that he would be moving in with a friend on MacDougal Street. As soon as he left, Nikos and I simultaneously whooped with delight. I could move in the next month. True, the five flights up, the roaches and the poor heating were all reminiscent of my hovel in Chicago, but I would have walked up ten flights just to be with this gorgeous creature. Anyway, Nikos's lease was up the end of April; then we would search for something more befitting a rich Greek and his Wall Street lover.

If sex were an Olympic event, Nikos would have won more gold medals than Mark Spitz. While my relationship with Bud had been based on romance, and with Keith, friendship and humor, with Nikos it was unabashed, passionate sex. For months we literally could not keep our hands off each other. We became known to friends as the Siamese twins. All I had to do was look into those hypnotic black pools of his eyes and I was silly putty in his hands. But besides the sex, I think the strength of our relationship was based on the attraction of opposites: the dark Mediterranean type and the blond Nordic type. This prevented the jealousy and insecurity found in most gay relationships, both by enhancing our mutual attraction and by reassuring each of us that when third parties admired one of us more than the other; it was not because of superior attractiveness, but rather a preference for that physical type. The result was, for both of us, a feeling of unprecedented security.

Unfortunately, our aesthetic tastes were just as opposite. This we discovered in the beginning of April when we moved into our new apartment and then set about furnishing it. The apartment we found was on the top floor of a beautiful old brownstone on the Seminary block of Chelsea: a large living room with brick wall and fireplace, bedroom also with fireplace and an enormous picture window framing a spectacular view of the Empire State and Chrysler buildings; the dream love nest.

But in furnishings, Nikos preferred New Wave and I, Americana. The two went together like ketchup and molasses. And self-centered as each of us was, compromise was difficult. But at the same time, I was determined not to jeopardize what could grow into a lifetime commitment over conflicting tastes in chatchkas. So we furnished the place in Nikos's postmodern, then I flew to Dubuque, rented a station wagon and brought back my folk art collection. Ketchup and molasses, perhaps, but on thick slices of domestic harmony.

I couldn't wait to show friends the idyllic life Nikos and I had created so we decided to have a party. Except for Nikos's souvlaki, neither of us knew how to boil an egg, much less whip up a salmon mousse. So we headed over to Dean and Deluca, the upscale and outrageously expensive grocer, and loaded up on caviar, ten bottles of Moet champagne, every kind of cheese ever made, shrimp, and pâté de foie gras. If it impressed the guests the way the bill impressed me, I could look forward to at least a dozen heart attacks; it came to $450. Holy quail brains, *I* couldn't afford that—but somehow Nikos could, and did. Was he a male prostitute? I was rather curious to know.

Mail the following day provided the answer to this unfathomable and vexatious mystery. Nikos's father, Stavros, had sent an $80,000 wire transfer from Swiss Bank Corp., Zurich, to Nikos's Citibank account.

Suffice it to say that this revelation did not diminish my feelings for Nikos in the slightest. If he was rich as well as gorgeous, I would just have to live with it.

We had invited thirty people, for nine o'clock. I couldn't wait to exhibit my new possession. Not my folk art—Nikos. I almost felt I should unveil him, like a flawless Greek statue. Pride of ownership.

At 9:30, not one soul had arrived. I sat on the couch, chain smoking and nail biting, wondering if we could return the food. Finally, at a quarter to ten the first guest arrived. It was José, an extremely sexy Cuban whom Nikos loathed because of his flirtations with me. Just like Nikos would do, I played it to the hilt, eating up the flattery with ravenous delight. I was the star and Nikos my accessory. Suddenly the doorbell began to ring off the wall. The thirty invited guests had nearly doubled. It became elbow to elbow and I began to fear that one of the drunken revelers would stumble into a delicate piece of folk art and turn it into kindling, or go shopping in my closet for an expensive leather jacket or cashmere sweater. Nevertheless, for the duration of the evening I was the consummate host. It was a matchmaker's dream: loads of beautiful men cruising for partners. That included José—with me as his target.

Meanwhile, Nikos began to get very friendly with every blond stud on the premises. That they appreciated him, too, was evident from certain discernible anatomical enlargements or swellings. I excused myself from José and joined Nikos in the midst of conversation with one of them. "What do you think, Jim?" Nikos whispered into my ear. "We can have him if we want." What I thought was, I didn't like it. But the *more* I thought, I thought, why not? The voyeur in me said, why not indeed? How sexy it would be to watch my beautiful Nikos interlocked with this blond bombshell.

But—but could I handle it? Or would jealousy head its ugly rear? Might Nikos fall in love with this guy and dump me? It was a tough decision, but I got paid to make tough decisions. I decided to go through with it. The erotic possibilities of a ménage à trois were irresistible. As the remaining revelers stumbled out, I retreated to the bedroom to disrobe and waited for Nikos and our friend to return with a vial of coke. As the stranger, Eric, sensuously peeled off his Calvin Klein underwear, a mammoth organ flopped out covering golf-ball-size testicles. Shit, Jim, what are you doing? You're going to lose Nikos if you go through with this. I glanced at Nikos for assurance there would be no threat, and whispered, "Safe only, Nikos, no swallowing cum, no fucking."

Nikos' eyes grew wide with ravenous lust and he was immediately down on the hardening cock, licking and sucking it like a giant candy cane. Suddenly Eric pulled his engorged member out of Nikos's mouth and began to finger his ass with some vaseline. I had to draw the line. "We're not into that, Eric, we want to remain safe." A disappointed Nikos turned around with begging eyes. "Nikos," I said, "if your little bung hole is hungry, why don't you feed it with a little Jimbo dick?" I straddled him doggy-style and began humping his tight hairy buns while our guest toyed with his uncut dick.

As far as the third guy went, it was a mutual satisfaction of each other's sexual hunger, no more, no less. As long as that was all he got from either of us—no romantic looks, no words of love—we knew we could handle it. From that night on it was agreed that we would be monogamous with the exception of an occasional third party for variety.

The onset of spring turned our thoughts toward Fire Island, the isle of iniquity. Nikos and a friend from the gym had discussed renting a house, and called a meeting to work out the details. There were eight of us altogether, an ad hoc combination of homos. Fred, a bartender at The Saint, had found a place on Fisherman's Walk at the far eastern end of the island for a measly $8,000 for the season. Half shares would be $1,000 per person. I could tell immediately that Nikos and I would never be bosom buddies with any of this motley crew; they were like a gaggle of old geese, arguing over everything from food to toilet paper. But the price was right.

The season started June 1 and Nikos and I were the first on the ferry from Sayville. As we pulled into the tiny harbor at the Pines, the island's gay capital, we smiled at each other in anticipation of the fantasy summer ahead. Upon disembarking, we rented a wagon, loaded it up with groceries and began our long trek down the wood plank walk to our house, which was little more than a two-story tree house on stilts. Thanks to an unlucky coin toss for the bedrooms, ours was the one downstairs, a dark, dank space with mold growing on the walls. Soon the other members started to straggle in. Christopher, a raving young prima donna, only seemed interested in shooting up heroin, and his skinniness and haggard eyes showed it. His friend Morgan, an obese, mustachioed queen who made jewelry for a living, was his partner in self-destruction.

"Oh, shit, Nikos, who have we gotten ourselves involved with?"

"Don't worry about it, Jim; we don't have to associate with them. There's a lock on our bedroom door and we'll just shut them out."

Eager to hit the beach and get tanned in preparation for our first night of dancing at the pavilion, I threw off my clothes, changed into my Speedo and giddily darted off with Nikos to peruse the bathing beauties in their oily glory. As Nikos and I walked west arm in arm, our egos were fed by all the heads we turned. I felt like yelling out, "Look at this hot stud that is all mine, you wimpy faggots; eat your hearts out." Why didn't I? I don't know.

We ran into Daniel, an Australian who worked in television production, and Bill, a blue-blooded Virginian real estate broker, both friends of mine from the old Studio days. They invited us to a white party on the beach, the first of countless theme parties of the summer.

Following about twenty feet behind Daniel was an emaciated, balding figure with so many purple KS tumors he looked like a human Dalmatian. I shuddered in fear, wondering if and when my rather liberal sexual past would catch up with me. If only I could turn back the clock. But would I have had the self-discipline, the willpower to abstain? Not likely. But at least now I had my one and only, and a mutual pledge of monogamy.

After our beach stroll we returned to our hovel to shower, smoke weed and fuck. Suddenly, Christopher, no doubt suffering from a drug hangover, screamed from upstairs, "Ease up, you assholes, you're going to shake the place off its foundation."

"Oh, eat shit and die, jerk," Nikos yelled back, and we burst into laughter. "Eat shit and die!" What a wit. We showered off the sex and went up to the kitchen for a drink and a shrimp cocktail before the tea dance. The trouble was — I hardly know how to put it, it was so disturbing and bizarre — *the shrimp was gone.* Suddenly Christopher walked in. What do you suppose he had hanging out of his mouth? Can't you guess? *A giant prawn.* I screamed, "You son of a bitch, Christopher, if you ever do anything like that again I'll beat the shit out of you." I mean, why *over*react? It was only his first offense. Cowering, the vicious little criminal darted out of the house and ran down the beach, no doubt looking for another fix.

Nikos and I spent the night dancing at the Pavilion. A full moon lit our way down the long wooden walkways. The sound of crashing waves mixed with the far-off beat of the disco. The mosquitos attacked without mercy. It was all so romantic. The club was an island version of The Saint, except instead of retreating to banquettes for breathers, it was just a short stumble to the beach to air out our sweat-soaked bodies. There in the dark, we could sit on the sand and drink in the balmy night air, or make love.

We spent the next day soaking up sun and exploring the quiet, shady walkways lined with Malibu-like houses at the far eastern end of the Pines. After a late afternoon tea dance we reluctantly boarded the ferry back to Sayville and the train into the city.

This was to be our rhythm throughout the long summer — idyllic weekends on Fire Island alternating with the unbearable heat and humidity of New York. Every weekday morning I would walk down 23rd Street to the subway at Seventh Avenue and wedge myself into one of the cattle cars for the lurching, clattering ride downtown, and stand stewing in the thick miasma of sweat, stench and anger through the interminable mid-tunnel stops; then walk the four blocks from the Wall Street station to Water Street amid a procession of bleary-eyed brokers and office workers preparing to face another day of dog-eat-dog dealing and intra-office scheming. What more could anyone want? Just kidding. All that sustained me was thinking about my next weekend with Nikos on Fire Island.

Especially coveted was the Fourth of July weekend, for which the sharers in the house scrambled and squabbled to reserve accommodations for lovers and friends. Late in the afternoon of the Fourth, Nikos and I joined the crowd around the dock of the Pines harbor for the traditional arrival of the "ferry of fairies" from Cherry Grove, a less tony gay haven about a mile down the beach. The boat full of drag queens pulled in and moored; off stepped Marilyn Monroes and Liza Minnellis and Ann Millers and Barbra Streisands, cheered by a cast of thousands.

In the middle of this madness, the well-known New York photographer Alex Biltmore approached Nikos and me and said, "Come on you two, I want to catch you before you lose it."

Unsure what to make of this, but flattered, we agreed to meet him at the end of the dock a half hour later; he wanted to shoot as the sun was beginning to set. Nikos and I scrambled back to the house to gather a few of our favorite tattered jeans and sweats and returned to the dock to find Alex waiting with his camera. Nikos, who quietly but clearly envied my short-lived modeling career, began making cliché "model" faces, much like I'd done on my first shoot. Alex directed him to relax and pretend he wasn't in front of a camera. A roll of film and a joint or so later, he finally loosened up. About ten days later, back in the city, Alex called and said he had a contact sheet ready to show us. We met him at his studio in the East Fifties, and the shots just blew us away. Apart from their artistic quality, Alex had captured what was to remain one of the happiest moments in my life. We had about half of them blown up and framed and hung over the fireplace in our bedroom. They made my treasured folk art collection seem worthless in comparison.

As summer ended we almost tearfully bid our island idyll a fond farewell and returned to the city for the long grey winter, consoling ourselves with thoughts of love-filled nights in front of the fireplace as the snow swirled outside.

Before the miseries and comforts of winter, however, summer had one last stand. Nikos and I went to Greece in early September. Touring the island with a beautiful Greek; who could possibly ask for more? After a fourteen-hour flight, we touched down in Athens around noon and were met by Nikos's parents: Eleni, a soft-spoken, elegantly dressed woman, and Stavros, who resembled Prince Rainier, and was probably in Greece what a Don was in Italy.

In the baking heat, we shuffled across the parking lot to Stavros's vintage Mercedes, then drove to Voulagmeni, an upscale suburban area where Nikos had a penthouse apartment overlooking the Mediterranean. After a delicious lunch of Greek salad, moussaka and baklava, Eleni and Stavros went back to their penthouse in the city, and Nikos and I headed across the street to go waterskiing. When Nikos finished showing off his championship skills and we headed back to shore, I noticed a beautiful young man whose equipment bulged through his skimpy swimsuit like an outboard motor. He was watching us admiringly from the dock.

"What do you think, Nikos?"

"I think he needs his hole worked out."

"I'm sure if anyone can do it you certainly can."

The young man approached and introduced himself; he was a Greek named Dominic. Nikos asked him up for a drink. In the elevator, Nikos slid his hand under Dominic's swimsuit to examine the merchandise, then gave me a little smiling nod. Inside, Nikos planted himself on the couch next to Dominic, then reached over and pulled his zipper down to uncover a monstrous piece of flesh which he immediately engulfed with his mouth. How sexy it was to see my lover with another hot man; a fantasy starring two Greek gods; mythology come to life. Nothing like this had happened my first day—or any—of my trip with Julio and David. But as I always said, the right place at the right time with the right people. Nikos was the right people. And maybe Greece was the right place.

Nikos's mother would be on her way back soon to cook dinner so we ushered Dominic out and bid him farewell. After we'd cleaned up the evidence, Sophia, a good friend of Nikos's and fellow NYU student, dropped in. The two of them were trying to figure out how to get the coveted U.S. green card. Suddenly, I had it.

"Nikos, how would you like to become my nephew?"

"I would love to, Jim. What are you talking about?"

"My niece is an au pair up in Ridgefield, Connecticut, and desperately wants to attend Parsons School of Design. Unfortunately my brother's divorce has sapped his financial resources. You'd have to pay her. It's worth a try. The only thing is that screwing around with your uncle is incestuous, you know."

"Do you have a nephew too, Jim?" Sophia asked.

"I do, but he's only fifteen and I don't think he's ready for a serious commitment."

Eleni arrived with the makings of a Greek feast—calamari, souvlaki, Greek salad and baklava. After putting away groceries, she offered to read my cards; it seemed she was an amateur fortune-teller. But the suggestion frightened me a little, as though somewhere in the back of my mind I knew it would not be good news. I respectfully declined.

The candle-lit dinner on Nikos's enormous terrace was the perfect cap to my first full day in Greece, despite the frustration of the language barrier. (There's nothing worse than sitting stonefaced while everyone laughs at jokes that you *know*, in your paranoia, are about you.) Stavros, knowing that I worked on Wall Street (I had been at Credit Suisse for over a year), questioned me about investment possibilities. He had been hit a couple of years before for a half million by the slump in gold prices, and wanted to be extra-careful. I wanted to say, "Why don't you invest in early American folk art?" But not every Greek tycoon appreciates fine, rotten old weather vanes.

The following day we battled through the heavy traffic free-for-all around the Plaka in central Athens on our way to the port of Piraeus to catch the ferry to the islands. Surprisingly, there were none of the German or Japanese tourists on board that I'd gotten used to seeing everywhere. The passengers were mostly native islanders: toothless, bowlegged old women dressed in black, carrying chickens in cages; one bedraggled old man actually brought on a goat which, unnerved by all the people, proceeded to take a big dump on the floor. The smell, combined with that of the passengers themselves and the rolling of the sea, would—I told myself as I leaned over the rail—remain one of my most vivid memories.

At five in the afternoon we docked at Nikos's mother's ancestral island of Tinos, where tourists were few and traditional ways still held sway. No sooner had we disembarked than I noticed three old, unshaven men in tattered, baggy black suits and suspenders. One Anthony Quinn-like figure got up out of his rickety chair, went over to a clothesline full of fresh squid hanging in the sun to dry, took one off, brought it over to the others as they poured three glasses of ouzo, cut the slimy thing up and swallowed it. So struck was I by this stark, elemental, almost primeval scene of Mediterranean life that it just took my appetite clean away.

Tinos could not have been more untouristy or unspoiled. Scattered about the island were over five hundred chapels, each more picturesque than the next, with their whitewashed walls and bell towers, with robin's egg blue domes. Life inched along at a snail's or squid's pace; the local yokels seemed to have made hanging out into an art; it was almost a Greek version of Andy Griffith's Mayberry. Nikos and I followed the street alongside the harbor to his mother's apartment. The place was almost monastically bare, with only a few sticks of furniture and none of the garish opulence of their apartment in Athens. I figured they kept the place to remind them both of what they had achieved in life, and what they had left behind.

The simplicity was all very wonderful, but my thoughts were upon the hedonistic pleasures that awaited us in Mykonos, just a forty-five minute ferry ride away. And on that ferry Nikos and I were the next afternoon, high in more ways than one — up on the top deck, smoking a joint, laughing giddily at Nikos's impersonation of a Greek whore, and soaking up the sun. Entering the harbor at Mykonos, we passed sleek yachts from all over Europe and fantasized about which jet setters and tycoons might own them, and what hot crewmen they might have in their employ. We found a quaint little guest suite two blocks from the harbor, dumped our bags, dropped magic mushrooms and were off on the maze of winding streets without a care in the world, darting in and out of boutiques and seaside tavernas. We strutted around, shirtless, ogling and being ogled, basking in all the ego-boosting attention. Sunset found us dining at the Gnosos, a cozy little rendezvous overlooking the Mediterranean. I stared across the table into Nikos's eyes and choked up with tears at my happiness. After dinner I took his hand and led him back to our suite to express my feelings for him in private. It was my twenty-seventh birthday, and Nikos informed me that all I had to do to get my present was to unzip his pants; and what a birthday gift it was. If only the moment could last forever; a beautiful Greek man, a romantic Greek island, and the whole night before us.

It was also the birthday of the owner of Filipe's, the hottest club in Mykonos, the ultimate jet set hangout; and as Nikos and I walked along the harbor to the club, ravishing young women were alighting from yacht launches on their way to the party in their Scassi, Herrera, Halston and Blass. We danced the night away shirtless. Unfortunately for the designer-clad women, all eyes seemed to be on us.

We returned to Athens the following week for our departure home. Upon arrival in New York I called my niece to propose our marriage brainstorm.

"Christi, I know you're dying to go to Parsons. I think I may have the solution. Nikos needs a wife to get his green card so he can work here in the U.S. You'd live with us for one year and divorce him once he gets the card. In return you'll receive a check for $5,000. Don't worry, it will be totally platonic. No one will ever know other than the three of us. You'd have to sign a premarital agreement, though." The deal was struck and Christi married Nikos and moved in the following week. My lover, my nephew-in-law; it was too much.

Back at the Credit Suisse office, a finance deal for a coal mining project in Kentucky was waiting on my desk. The following week my yuppie colleague Jeffrey and I left for an overnight trip to the site. Clothed in full mining gear we descended hundreds of feet into the earth to four-foot-high tunnels where a giant scraper deposited coal onto a conveyer system to be carried out of the mine. Jeffrey sweated profusely, apparently from a touch of claustrophobia. After a full day of crawling around like gophers, we returned to the Holiday Inn with aching muscles. Jeffrey offered me a back rub, straddled me and began. Soon his hands gravitated towards my crotch and I flushed with embarrassment at the uncomfortable situation. "Thanks, Jeffrey, I think I've had enough." So I was right about Jeffrey. I'd suspected he was a closet case; he periodically made mysterious trips to the Village to meet "a friend"; besides, he simply had too much style not to be. Well, be that as it may, there was one mineshaft he would not be exploring.

My first autumn and holiday season with Nikos brought its memorable moments. We went to the Halloween party at The Saint, he as a devil—appropriately—in black tights, red sequined horns, tail and pitchfork, and cowboy boots from his Imelda Marcos-sized collection, sprayed red; and I as an angel—*not* so appropriately—in white tights, glitter wings, halo and a sequined wand. We were the hit of the ball. At Christmas, I brought Nikos home to my parents. My mother, strangely enough, offered us their bedroom suite. If she had known what went on in her bed she'd probably have wanted to have me castrated.

After our return, Christi's presence became more and more of a burden. We were trapped for the most part in our bedroom, carefully suppressing our sound effects during sex. Spacious as the apartment was by New York standards, it was beginning to become claustrophobic and tensions between Nikos and me grew. Some nine months later, Nikos got a call to set up the dreaded Immigration interview. Christi seemed amazingly relaxed, but Nikos was a nervous wreck. Each had to be familiar with the most minute detail regarding the other; we had been told that one never knew what kind of trick questions might pop up. I was the coach, dreaming up possible questions.

"Christi, this might be embarrassing, but it's something you must know, just in case. Nikos is uncircumcised. And you use prophylactics; children are not in your plans for the immediate future."

Christi looked away, blushing. Okay, so maybe those weren't the first questions they'd ask. But you could never know what kind of pervert of an inspector you might draw.

On the morning of the interview, *I* was a nervous wreck. I could lose my lover, my niece would be calling my brother, sobbing and begging him to get her out of jail, and I would be disowned. I sat in my office, waiting for their call, chain-smoking and shuffling papers in a neurotic semblance of working. When I spilled my coffee on my morning mail, Bruce, a fellow officer, said, "For Christ's sake, what is the matter with you today? You look like you're on a speed trip."

I couldn't very well explain the situation. "It's just this Greek bombshell I've been seeing. I think she might be out whoring around on me."

"Get over it. This is New York City. There's plenty of fish in the sea, and I'm sure you could sack any one of them if you wanted." Thanks, Bruce, I'll keep that in mind.

At last my phone rang. "Success! Alright!" I yelled. Everyone in my department turned their heads, thinking I had just bagged a deal. Which, of course, I had.

Chapter 12

The Big A

While the sick man has life, there is hope.

—Cicero

There are no such things as incurables; there are only things for which man has not found a cure.

—Bernard M. Baruch

That October, 1985, I began to notice that I didn't seem to have the strength I'd always had, and I looked peaked and washed out. Being a former model, I knew that blonds tend to age, appearance wise, at a younger age than darker people; I mean, look at Lena Horne. But Christ, I was only 28. Was it already time for Geritol? I was also having unusual difficulty getting my spread sheets to reconcile at work. I couldn't lift as much at the gym, and my sexual vigor and activity were diminished. I feared that Nikos was turning elsewhere, and tensions grew between us. Who was he having sex with? Well, himself, for one—that much I knew: We now slept in separate beds—or I should say, I slept while he spent the whole night out in the living room, satiating his desires with a ten-inch dildo, a vial of coke and porno movies on the video recorder. Periodically I would call out to him to come to bed. I would wake up in the morning and there he was, going for the Guinness Book of World Records. It was surprising that he had any rectum left, the way he was going with that piece of plastic.

We had one more happy time together: After much debate, we went back to Greece, this time taking in Santorini, the most beautiful of all the islands, with its whitewashed, blue-domed buildings clinging to the edge of the cliffs. In Athens, once again Nikos's mother served us a fabulous Greek feast of calamari, moussaka and lamb. Again, she brought out her cards and insisted on telling my future, and again I vehemently declined, sensing somehow that the death card would come up.

During the trip I also noticed what seemed to be a loss in short-term memory, evidenced by lost wallets, sunglasses and keys; and some loss of coordination in things like waterskiing.

In February of the following year a purple lesion appeared on my nose. At first I wrote it off as just another zit, but when it still had not healed a month later, I became worried and called Nikos's doctor, John Montana, who recommended Mary Ellen Bradamus, a dermatologist and wife of the president of Columbia University. Dr. Bradamus seemed concerned and wanted to do a biopsy; oh, God, no, she's going to cut into my nose. Without anesthesia, she yanked a tissue sample out, leaving me covered with blood and in excruciating pain. The results came back after a week of sleepless nights. Mary Ellen brought me into her office, sat me down and dropped the bombshell of my life.

"Jim, I don't know how to easily break the news to you, but it's been diagnosed as Kaposi's sarcoma. You have AIDS."

The denial stage had come to a crashing end, landing in devastating reality. There were no tears, just bitterness for the beautiful, perfect life that had suddenly been pulled from beneath me.

Now I had to face Nikos and my family with the news. I returned home and, finding Nikos in his usual position in front of the VCR, I flew into a rage, screaming and sobbing, and threw the VCR down the stairs. He was speechless. His face turned white and sullen. He knew. A week went by and not a word was spoken.

As little as I wanted to be associated with anything AIDS related, I figured I should try a support group. I found one which was held in the crumbling, smelly basement of a brownstone in Greenwich Village. At this point I was too weak to handle the subway, so Jeffrey gave me a stack of car vouchers on the pretext that I had a liver disease. How long I could carry on such pretenses, I didn't know.

A group of about fifteen sat on stained, smelly furniture around the perimeter of the room. Each person seemed more bizarre than the next: The man next to me weighed about 350 pounds; he was covered with tattoos and dressed in black leather vest and pants, and made S&M jewelry for a living; the girl next to him was a pasty-faced drug addict with a purple Mohawk hairdo, who babbled about her various hocus-pocus homemade remedies. I was in the middle of a circus freak show. Did I now belong with this trash?

The discussion went around the room as one by one they poured out their souls, describing their attempts to deal with the disease. When my turn came, I stood up and did nothing but stutter for about three minutes. I could not form a single sentence. I thought my brain had come apart; a complete nervous breakdown. Terrified, I ran out of the building and started walking in what I thought was the direction home, only the surroundings looked unfamiliar. Straight ahead was the World Trade Center; I was lost in an area just blocks from my apartment. Thank God I had my wallet with me with my driver's license, otherwise I'd probably still be wandering around lower Manhattan. I grabbed a cab home and called my doctor, who explained that it was just a temporary chemical imbalance, that my brain was fine but that disorientation might occur from time to time.

Now I had to make the dreaded call to my parents—and it would be a double whammy. Mother had always asked, "When are you going to bring home the right girl?"

"When the right girl has a sex change," I had always felt like replying. Instead I said, "Mother, all you should be concerned with is my happiness, and I'm happy." But I think she suspected that something wasn't right ever since she caught me in her makeup drawer and trying on her wigs as a youth.

I dialed the number with a lump in my throat. "Mother, are you sitting down? I've got some bad news to tell you. I've been diagnosed as having AIDS." Silence. At that moment I was no longer her pride and joy. I was a disgrace. The golden boy had instantaneously metamorphosed into the black sheep. I had tried all my life to make my parents proud of me, to fulfill every dream they had for me, and it had all been in vain. I could hear the sobs on the other end. "Where did we fail you? How could you ever have become so perverse?"

"Mom, to me my sexual preference is only that. I'm not a fag, sissy or queen, I'm still the same Jimmy you've always loved. To me, my sexuality has always been as simple as a preference for chocolate over vanilla ice cream. At least I've experienced love. Many people never do. I've no regrets. I kept this thing a secret all my life for fear of being disowned. Believe me, it's been no picnic leading a double life. I love you with all my heart. Please don't abandon me, Mother.'' She was on a plane the next day.

Nikos then dropped another bombshell: He was leaving me. Begging him in tears to stay with me through this thing, I reminded him, in vain, of that solemn promise we had made to each other years ago, that if one of us got it, the other would be there for him.

I greeted Mother at the door in sobs. Then we hit the classifieds in search of a small studio; alone, I couldn't afford the $1,500 a month Nikos and I were paying. Finding something affordable in New York was a horror story for anyone, but being dragged around the city when you can barely make it up the stairs was almost too much. I couldn't go home to Iowa to live out my remaining days; the medical treatment available in Sundown Town wouldn't be as good, and my parents and I would drive each other crazy.

The whole housing hunt is a vague blur in my memory, but I do remember that it seemed as if half the places we tried to see either didn't exist or no one came by to show them. The affordable possibilities we did see were quite a comedown from the Chelsea brownstone, and a hospice was definitely out: No way would I surround myself with a bunch of end-stagers. Finally, we took a brand new ninth-floor studio on 19th Street, two blocks south of the brownstone. Mother thought it lovely. I thought it more generic than a box of corn flakes. Its only selling point was a large picture window view of the Chrysler and Empire State buildings, the same view as from Nikos's and my old bedroom. Moving my belongings was probably the most painful thing I'd ever done in my life. The finality of my separation from Nikos was almost too much to bear.

What with my reduced motor skills and my bereaved state of mind, while moving a rare piece of folk art — a flying-duck decoy — I accidentally broke the wing. Devastated, I called Kelter-Malcé, a dealer on Bleeker Street, and asked about the possibility of restoring the piece. They recommended a Jane Pfersdorf, who had previously worked at the Metropolitan Museum but now had her own restoration business, and whose expertise ran the gamut from pre-

Columbian to old masters. I took the piece to her workshop loft in the Times Square area.

Wiry and intense, Jane was the quintessential Renaissance woman. As we talked, my bladder, its endurance diminished by my illness, suddenly demanded relief. Jane directed me to the curtained-off end of the loft. I pushed the curtain aside, and beheld a masterpiece: a large, late 19th-century Italian oil painting of an aging, fat and pathetically lonely-looking woman sitting on a rickety chair, a wilted rose lying across her loins symbolizing her unplucked and never-to-be-plucked virginity. My rose had been plucked long ago, I reflected, but my future prospects for sexual fulfillment were now no better than hers.

When I came back out I asked Jane about the painting. She explained that a man had come in with a very intricate, ancient Mayan piece that needed restoring before he put it up for sale as part of a divorce settlement. As payment for her work, Jane had accepted the painting. She showed me crackled old newspaper clippings describing the anonymous work as equalling or exceeding in quality the great Renaissance masters.

I guessed that she needed money more than an art collection, and would probably sell for the right price. Playing on the fact that I had AIDS and that my financial future was as uncertain as my life, I invoked my still intact Wall Street shmoozing techniques, swallowed a frog in my throat, and made an offer of $3,500. Jane was struggling visibly over whether to give up her treasure. In good divorce-settlement spirit, I offered full visitation rights, and promised her the picture's bequest in the event of my death. At last Jane's pained look gave way to a smile; she said it would give her no greater personal satisfaction than to bring some joy into my stricken life. Thus began a friendship that kept growing steadily, into eternal, unconditional love. God, what I had missed in life by sacrificing what is really meaningful for the sake of the frivolous, the merely physical, the short-lived! If only I had not been possessed by this evil homosexual lust, Jane would have been prime life-partner material.

At work, I made it clear to everyone that the spots on my nose were the result of a liver disease. I tried my best to cover up my lesions by using everything from Clearasil to Clinique, but everything seemed to be absorbed on contact. Finally, at a follow-up meeting with beautiful Mary Ellen (Dr. Bradamus), she suggested a cover-up product by Lydia O'Leary that former model-slash-victim Marla Hansen was touting. What was harder to hide was that I had ballooned up to 198 pounds; In my depression I was back gorging on two pints of Haagen Dazs a night.

Work itself became more and more difficult. There was a lull in the market and borrowings were down severely. However, public and private finance deals were booming, and lucite "tombstones" from *The Wall Street Journal*—the trophies for these deals—seemed to pour in daily. I decided on my own to prospect some real estate participations and was thrilled to get a shot at 900 North Michigan Avenue, a $500 million multi-use skyscraper to be built in Chicago. Plans for tenants included a Four Seasons hotel, Plitt theaters, condos, and office space, and Bloomingdale's had committed to a new store. How impressive to be included in the bank consortium that brought Bloomie's to Chicago. Wouldn't Bud reel!

But my ability to do my job was deteriorating by the minute. Goldman Sachs, one of the bank's most coveted clients, called to renew a $50 million letter of credit. The credit line renewal package was nowhere near completion and I had to inform them that they'd have to look elsewhere. Outraged at our inability to accommodate, Kirsten, a VP in Goldman's treasury department, called Jeffrey to complain. The gig was up. I was immediately called into his office to explain. Trembling, I informed him of my diagnosis, and at the same time pleaded with him for his OK to start prospecting real estate development companies, in view of my getting the 900 North Michigan Avenue deal. Instead, Jeffrey yanked all my accounts and assigned me to Chris O'Connell, a geeky, pasty-faced AVP who sat behind me and seemed to talk about nothing but his new baby boy. I hated his blond guts and cringed whenever he ordered me to do something.

Promotions were imminent and I reminded Jeffrey that a year before he had promised me my AVP title. I had done a great job, taking full responsibility for developing from scratch a $750 million loan portfolio with major brokers, dealers and investment banks. I made it clear that I felt he had lied to me about my promotion.

"YOU'RE FIRED! YOU'RE FIRED!" he yelled. Dumbstruck,

I could only stare at the lucite "tombstone" of the announcement for 900 North Michigan Avenue on his desk.

"Please, Jeffrey, don't do this. Please, Jeffrey."

"Jim, why don't you go on disability? You'll get sixty percent of your salary and your insurance pays a hundred percent of your medical bills. Retire."

"Because I love my job and I love working. I can do it."

"You can't. I've got a list three pages long of your fuck-ups."

"I'd like to see it."

"Only when you quit."

I shuffled out of his office to my desk, and left soon after. First my lover was gone, now my job. I wanted to make sure all the i's were dotted and t's crossed before I asked for my disability papers, so I decided to get an attorney. I called Doug Curtis, a good friend and Vice President in the legal department at Morgan Guaranty, who suggested Trevor Roland, a Harvard-trained whiz kid. Roland was on his way to Europe, but said he would be happy to take my case upon his return. Then I called my mother to tell her this latest news.

"Oh, no, Jimmy, how can you do this? How will you live?"

"Mother, the emotional pain is just too much. My brain has been affected by this disease. The numbers are just too difficult to work. Last week I forgot to renew Goldman's credit line and we lost a hundred thousand dollars in income, not to mention jeopardizing the account. Jeffrey just made it clear there was no future for me there and requested I resign."

"But what will you do?"

"Liquidate all that I have and buy and sell folk art."

I could tell her heart was broken. She had tearfully told her bridge club about my AIDS; now it was all over town. If only she could have bit her tongue, or said cancer. How could I ever hold my head up in Sundown Town again?

The last thing I wanted was to end up in some hospital on my deathbed not having done the things I'd always wanted to do, which included sailing in Nantucket and driving around Maine in the peak of the leaf season to hunt for antiques. Another was getting my religion in order, so I began classes at Trinity Church in preparation for conversion to Episcopalianism. I realized, looking back over my life, that getting my wings might prove a little harder than it had been dressing up as an angel for Halloween, but I thought it certainly worth a try. At least I believed in God. Twice a week I would go to noontime mass and a healing service immediately following where a small line would form in the chancelry and each congregant would approach the priest at the altar. My first time, the priest, a short, elderly, ex-Wall Street banker with the most serene and genuinely concerned expression, gently placed his hands on my shoulders and spoke.

"And what can I do for you, son?"

I explained my situation and he put his hands on my head and extemporized the most beautiful speech just for me. I felt as if God had shot through my body, and I was moved to tears.

My attorney finally got back from Europe and I met with him to get the OK—along with a bill for $800 for dime store legal work (which is exactly what I wrote on the check).

The following day I dropped into personnel to pick up the papers. On the way up in the elevator I ran into Jeffrey.

"Well, Jeffrey, you've got your wish. I just got the papers."

"How much did you settle for?"

"The sixty percent."

"I'll see if we can get you more. I think you've made the right decision. When are you leaving?"

"The usual two weeks."

"You can leave tomorrow. We'll pay you full salary through the end of the month. Just be sure you give instructions to Bill."

The next day I packed my personal belongings in cardboard boxes and called a bank limo to pick me up. The departure was anticlimactic, with no fanfare. It was to be made clear that I was leaving to pursue folk art.

Two weeks later Jeffrey called to invite me to lunch. I arrived at the office to find that he had rented a private dining room at Harry's, the bankers' old boys' club, which he knew was my favorite place to take clients, and that he had ordered Beef Wellington—my favorite dish—and five bottles of Moet. My entire department of fifteen came. I was overwhelmed. After thinking I would take leave of my career shunned and disgraced, this was totally unexpected. They insisted I sit at the head of the table, and made toasts to me. I toasted them back chokingly as the greatest group of people I'd ever worked with in my life.

I arrived home to find a message on my machine from Dr. Montana.

"They found a treatment, Jim. Burroughs Wellcome has developed AZT, a very strong antiviral which stops viral replication."

"Oh, thank God."

"I'll call in the prescription and you can pick it up this afternoon. Dosage is two pills every four hours around the clock."

After two weeks of the medicine I felt thoroughly and totally rejuvenated and the mirror no longer reflected death warmed over. In fact, I had more energy than I wanted: insomnia set in, and after weeks of sleepless nights I had to be given a prescription for Halcion, which put me out in five minutes. As a side effect of the AZT, however, neuropathy began to develop; it felt like I was being stuck by a hundred pins in my extremities, and there was nothing I could do about it.

The following month Nikos left for Greece where he would be tested.

The first of three auctions of the remainder of my folk art collection was held at Christie's soon afterwards. Cindy Weston, my old MHT Company training program buddy, had bought the best of my collection and it pleased me that someone I loved so dearly would be caretaker of my prized possessions. It was as if I was following in the footsteps of Jon Murray and his glass collection. The pre-auction estimates were fair and actual bids were both high and low. After the auction, as I was heading up Madison Avenue to look around in my favorite shops, I ran into my old St. Olaf roommate Lon Larsen, dressed head to toe in Armani. This was quite a step up from his Norwegian sweaters and clogs; no doubt the influence of his Italian boyfriend, Dodo.

"Well, Lon, how the hell ya doin'?"

Flustered at this unexpected meeting, he nervously fumbled with his Ferragamo clutch and choked on his words, obviously still feeling guilty over the dirty deed he had done me at school.

"Heard you have an Italian lover. That's great! I know how much we Scandinavians like those swarthy Mediterraneans. They're great in bed. Love to meet him." Lon turned red, but surprisingly made no attempt at denial. I walked away feeling at least partly avenged.

My nose lesions had grown to the point that they were impossible to hide. I looked like a disfigured Karl Malden. It was like having "AIDS" branded across my face. I couldn't go anywhere without the fear of people pointing in disgust. Mother and Dad sent me a plane ticket to come home to Dubuque for the spring to help me recoup. Once there, I became very nostalgic. I went through my old high school year books, and even invited an old teacher out for a drink. He was exactly as I remembered him, with his flawless sense of humor.

Mother was refusing to hear any discussion of my relationship with Nikos. She groaned in disgust as I brought out my prized book of photos of Nikos and me on the beach in Fire Island. Amazingly, my father, the consummate man's man, had little or nothing to say about my sexual preference; but mother began to rag on me for every little thing. My brother and I suggested she see a psychologist. It was clear she thought she had failed and it hurt me to no end to hear her lying on her bed sobbing. I had destroyed any chance of happiness in her golden years.

I invited an old childhood friend out for dinner. She had always been a tomboy and now taught literature at the Catholic High School. With her short-cropped hair and blue-tinted glasses, and all her friends being nuns, I figured she had to be a lesbian.

"Now that you know my story, why don't you tell me yours?"

She blushed deeply. "Jimmy, I'm still a virgin."

"Do you mean to tell me you've never been in love with a woman? Don't let love pass you by. It's part of life, and not to be missed. It's a gift from God." It was obvious that her devout Catholic Dubuque upbringing had stifled her emotionally; an acknowledgement of her true feelings would surely result in fire and brimstone.

With all my new-found energy, I wanted to swim laps in the Country Club pool, but without the little kids flopping around. I was on good terms with the club manager, Paul. "Sure, Jimmy," he said, "I'll just leave the gate open and you can swim to your heart's content." I was swimming, feeling like I was back on the swim team in high school, when all of a sudden there was my father up at the gate, motioning to me with his finger.

"Come on, Jimmy, get out. We don't want people to think you're contaminating the pool."

"Dad, you've got to be kidding."

"No, I'm not. Listen, we have to live here and people around here simply aren't educated as to how this disease is transmitted."

I felt leprous, but I respected my father enough to come out of the pool where I had not only lifeguarded but *saved* lives. I returned home and went out on the patio to do something about my sickly pallor and contemplate the horror of what had just occurred. It was a beautiful breezy day and my mind was wandering. Suddenly, I had the first of what would be many ESP experiences. Somehow I knew that Rob Seaver, one of my best friends, who had lived in the same apartment building as Chad and I, had died.

Upon my return to New York there was a rare message from Chad on my machine. "Hey, Jim, this is Chad. Give me a call."

I couldn't get ahold of him and called our mutual friend, Rick Webster.

"Rick, did Rob die of AIDS?"

"How did you know?"

"I don't know how I knew, I just did. Scary isn't it? He was my best friend."

Depressing as that was, it was time to proceed with my travel plans. My first trip would be sailing in Nantucket. I took the Carey bus out to La Guardia to find that the flight had been canceled due to fog. I had to sit around for a couple of hours to see if they were going to reschedule another or wait till the following morning. While having a sandwich at the airport Arby's, I was approached by a young black girl with a gold tooth and tattered clothing, who asked me for $2.69. Taken aback, I asked, almost laughing, "Why $2.69?"

"'Cause that's what the fried chicken costs."

I smiled, took out five dollars and told her to get something to drink and some dessert and asked her to come sit with me. She introduced herself as Jenny Moses, and told me that begging for money at the airport was the only way she could support her heroin habit and that she was being evicted from a welfare hotel in down-town Newark.

"Listen, sweetheart, you are a lovely young woman. You seem intelligent. You've got to get yourself off this shit. I'm going to say a big prayer for you tonight. Drugs are only a temporary escape. You always have to come back to reality." Then I told her about my condition. Her eyes welled up and she said she would pray for me as well.

They did not schedule another flight, so I hopped back on the Carey bus with a smile on my face, happy about helping the poor waif with something to eat and a few hopefully inspiring words.

Nikos had been gone for an inordinate amount of time. Still shaken by Rob's death, I had this horrible feeling that Nikos had tested positive and decided to take his own life. That night I made countless calls to Greece to no avail.

The next morning I headed back to the airport and caught an early flight. Once on the beautiful island I parked myself at a charming little bed and breakfast complete with a fireplace in my room, then rented a Jeep CJ7 to drive around the island and on the beach. As I drove by the harbor I noticed a sign advertising a three-hour sail cruise around the island. I took it, and it was on that cruise, while thinking back over my life, that I decided to write it all down. That's it, it would be my baby. My permanent mark on the world. My legacy. It would be the most challenging undertaking of my life. I began immediately, and with the stimulus of wind, sun, sails and water, words poured out like Niagara.

The autumn chill set in early in New York that year, but the landlord would not turn on the heat until the outside temperature was fifty or below. I bought a space heater which seemed to do the trick. But one particularly cold, windy, rainy, nasty night, I turned on the space heater, and soon started sweating profusely. I took my temperature: 103°. I opened the windows and applied a cold compress to my forehead. My sweat turned to a deathly chill. I panicked, fearing it was the beginning of the end. I called 911 and went down to the lobby to wait for an ambulance. When it finally got there I explained my condition to the loutish driver and his equally ill-mannered assistant, and said it was my first time in an ambulance.

"Well ya better get used to it buddy, 'cause this will be the first of many for you."

The inhumanity of the remark made me seethe. I got to St. Vincent's Hospital and they wheeled me into a very busy emergency room, laid me on a table and left me for over an hour, not even so much as taking my temperature. Finally I started to feel better and decided to just get up and go home. In my terror I had forgotten to bring my wallet, so I asked an intern and a nurse if I could borrow five dollars for cab fare.

"Take a bus." The bus did not go near my apartment, so I bundled up and set out in the raging storm to walk home. I got home drenched. I undressed, made myself a hot bubble bath and wrote a letter of complaint to St. Vincent's refusing to pay for services not rendered.

In the middle of October I purchased tickets for Jane and me to go to Maine. At the last minute she canceled because she had deadlines to meet for pieces she was restoring for the Fall Antique Show at the Pier; but her assistant Claire agreed to go in her place.

On the Carey bus to Newark we got stuck in a bumper-to-bumper jam. Watching the time tick by, it didn't look as if we were going to make it. We arrived at the very moment of our scheduled takeoff time and dashed off to our gate, O. J. Simpson-style. As we entered the security check I suddenly heard, "Bobby, Bobby." I turned around to find Jenny Moses, the girl with the gold tooth, now dressed in a blue blazer with name tag and a beige skirt. She had obviously forgotten my name but had gotten a job. "Alright! Go for it!" I yelled joyfully without stopping. Miracles do happen; I only hoped Jenny's prayer for me would work as well.

Upon arrival we rented a Chevy Citation, headed into Portland, checked in at a generic hotel and found a restaurant that served the famous Maine lobster. Two five-pounders for six dollars; amazing. The waitress, looking like Flo out of *Alice*, attached a ridiculously kitschy bib around my neck. An old lobster pro like me.

After our feast we headed across the street to Lobster Louie's Lounge for a drink. The interior was covered with fish nets, lobster baskets and tacky plastic lobsters hanging from the ceiling. We sat at the bar next to one Bertha Mae Pritchard, a lady of the night who had seen better and slimmer days. She was poured into a tight sequined T-shirt that barely covered her twenty-gallon jugs, a pair of designer jeans, and white stiletto heels, and was on the make with a fat truck driver wearing a farmer cap. The evening's crowning touch of tackiness occurred when a would-be Elvis lounge lizard in a polyester leisure suit came on, along with a piano accompanist, loosened his tie and launched into a pitiful rendition of "Blue Suede Shoes." Sated with local culture and one too many scotches, we finally stumbled out into the cold, damp Maine night.

I set the alarm for the crack of dawn so we could get to Kennebunkport and eat breakfast before the antique show started. It was of paramount importance to be the first in to view the choicest merchandise before it was snatched up.

The atmosphere was like a fire sale at Bloomie's. When the door opened, frenetic treasure hunters literally ran down the aisle. The first piece that caught my eye was a nearly four-foot, 1930s birdhouse, an exact replica of a New England church. I negotiated the price with the dealer and was ecstatic at the potential profit I could realize back in the city. Then I talked to a dealer from Pennsylvania and told her of my interest in Amish quilts. She said she had a very rare circle pattern out in her van, so we went out to see it. The design was so bold and fresh-looking, it was almost postmodern; another folk art coup.

Next, it was off to Bar Harbor. The leaves were like fireworks on the trees. Between my watching the scenery and scouting for weather vanes, it was a miracle that we and the car stayed in one piece. Suddenly to my right, on top of an old carriage house, I spotted a weathered wooden arrow with a carved acorn finial. I floored the brakes and fishtailed to a stop. Poor Claire — her nerves were getting hopelessly frazzled. Her idea of autumn was to walk around leaf hunting and contemplating nature. I must confess, I was driving the poor girl to tears with my frantic folk art pursuits. But I tried to compensate by picking up the tab for everything. What she had to understand was that I was determined to squeeze every last drop out of my suddenly shortened life.

I was now considering moving to Los Angeles, and realized I was going to have to drum up some money. So, back in New York, I called a dealer, Dan Edwards, and baited him with my pieces by the great woodcarver Albert Zahn. Dan brought many weather vanes to Jane who would add a crackled gilt finish to simulate aging and weathering, which doubled their value; a classic example of the "caveat emptor" setup.

He came over the following Monday and glanced around the room. "I'll take this, this, and that: $10,500. The Tree of Life, how do you know it's a Zahn?" I had my concocted story down pat: Some naive farmer had approached me at an auction in Milwaukee. He'd seen me buy a small carving of a man sitting on a pig holding a fishing pole baited with a corn cob. He told me he had noticed "woodcarvings" in the auction offering in the paper, and thought he could unload some stuff he had inherited from his uncle. I followed him out to his pickup, expecting nothing but junk, but was confronted by these fabulous carvings which I recognized as similar to ones pictured in the *National Book of American Folk Sculpture*. I instantly knew I had a major find. I felt like an archeologist discovering King Tut's tomb.

Dan bought that, and the piece. And I certainly bought his offer — in fact, I was overwhelmed. "Dan," I asked, "it's none of my business, but the BMW, the country house, daughter in expensive private school — do you have other business interests or family money?"

"Nope, I'm not even a collector. The only thing I collect are deposit tickets."

"Well, Dan, you are truly an inspiration. Let me shake your hand. You know, the New York dealers can be a bunch of backstabbers, but I want you to consider me a friend and colleague."

Gone were the policeman whirligig, the Tree of Life and the family of angels. I'd sworn I'd never sell them, but from now on I couldn't let emotional attachments get in the way of doing business.

The following week in New York was the big week of the year for Americana: the Fall Antique Show at the Pier and auctions at Christie's, Sotheby's and Doyle's. I bought a fifty-dollar preview ticket for the show and was one of the first there. Bursting with adrenalin I ran down the aisles scoping out everything from Homer and Jacobsen to Windsor chairs, samplers, and Amish quilts. One booth offered an early nineteenth-century red and white candy-striped barber pole, set into a base with inset panels of navy with white stars. It screamed Americana; I could almost hear Sousa striking up the band. I expected the price to be $10,000 or more, but it was a mere $2,500, and with bargaining and a dealer discount I got it down to $2,000. A month later it sold for over $4,000 at a Sotheby's auction. Ah, turning a profit—the best kind of Americana of all.

Next I ran over to the booth of a Madison Avenue toy dealer and sold him my steamship model, a piece he had long coveted, for $3,500. He was a flamboyant, touchy-feely queen in a silk blouson, constantly humming in a Tiny Tim falsetto, who did appraisals for my fine arts insurance policy for free and who had made it obvious since the day I met him that he coveted me as well. This is the only kind of piece you'll get from me, I thought as he wrote out the check.

It was the day before Halloween and I had arranged a birthday dinner for eight at the Odeon for Sterling Richardson, a friend from the old Studio days who was flying in from North Carolina. I had ordered a cake for the occasion and had "Reunion, the Geritol Club, Happy Birthday, Sterling" lettered on it. The group included a famous playwright, his artist lover, Bill Wallace and his roommate Billy. At one point during the meal I noticed Billy discreetly bring out a pill box and take two AZTs. God, is there no end to this scourge?

Sterling showed up just when dinner had ended. He was grandiose and braggadocious as ever: He apologized for being late due to a lengthy round of appointments with a roster of Fortune 500 companies that were all dying to get him to work for them. I looked across the table at Bill, and rolled my eyes; he returned a knowing smirk. Then Sterling informed us that his family had just sold their business for big bucks. "Jimmy, you're looking at a man who doesn't have to work. I'm off to see the world." I told Sterling how lucky he was, and that I had never had a birthday party in my life since it fell at the time of year when everybody was starting school.

"Jimmy, I'm going to throw the greatest party imaginable for you next year. I'm gonna fly everyone down to Charlotte and we'll have hot air balloons, caterer, and the whole bit."

"Sure, Sterling. I think you're probably full of more hot air than your balloons. Can I hold you to it?"

"Sure, Jim, I'm a man of my word."

"Okay, everybody, you're all witnesses." I couldn't help thinking that planning my funeral might be more appropriate than a birthday party.

After dinner, Sterling and I shared a cab uptown. "Sterling, please don't take offense, but why would you want to alienate everyone with your bragging?"

"Jimmy, I've applied to every large corporation in the country to no avail. It's just my nature to be grand."

"I know, Sterling, but it's hardly what you'd call endearing."

I entered my apartment to find my answering machine blinking. It was Nikos. Thank God, he's alive. My prayers were answered.

The following night, Halloween, I was to meet Sterling and a friend in the Village for the annual costume parade. I had bought an evil-looking, full-head punk rocker mask with bloodshot eyes and rubber Mohawk. I was planning to wear it with black spandex tights and a psychedelic, skin-tight wet suit vest. I asked Nikos over to get his reaction, expecting envy of, if not praise for, my creativity. He disappointed me.

"Jim, do you really want to wear that? Let's face it, neither one of us looks like he used to."

I felt crushed, but painful as it was to hear, he was right. I looked like a stuffed sausage. In my depression the foodaholic in me had reemerged; I was continuing to down two pints of Haagen Dazs a night and was tipping the scales at 196. I decided baggy khakis and an oversized sweatshirt would be, well, more fitting.

As always, the parade offered a visual feast. It was amazing that the somnambulistic drones I'd see on the way to work could be so imaginative in their costumery. Streets in the Village were closed to traffic, and as on New Year's Eve, people were out to cut loose from their stifling inhibitions. After the parade, Sterling asked me to tag along with him to a loft party in Soho. Guests included José, the Cuban beauty boy, whose interest in me Nikos resented so; Nelson, Rollerama's sexy skater extraordinaire and an ex-twirl of Nikos's, as well as a host of Fire Island studs. Not surprisingly, none of them expressed the least bit of interest in me with my extra poundage and dark-circled eyes.

When the party was over we headed for The Saint. Sterling had some "ecstasy" and I asked him for a toot. "Jim," he said, "I really don't think you should." So he knew. God, why couldn't I maintain my anonymity with this miserable disease? The few friends whose confidentiality I had trusted had failed me. Everyone knew. I felt as if they were all pointing at me, avoiding me like the plague. Suddenly I saw Nikos ridiculously dressed as a bumblebee and flirting with some blond hunk. I departed for home, alone, with painful memories of what was and would never be again.

The following morning Nikos called to tell me he had gotten his test results and they were negative. Thank God, that prayer at least was answered.

"Nikos, I quit my job and am thinking of moving to L.A. The medical care there is supposed to be the best in the country and the weather is always great. You don't want me anymore and I want to establish a new life, however short it may be."

"Are you sure you know what you're doing, Jim?"

"Why should I continue to pay nine seventy-five a month for this generic studio, vegging out, watching soaps and gorging myself on Haagen Dazs? I'm headed out the end of the week to see if I like it. I'll stay with Steve and Ernie. Why don't we get together for breakfast at the Empire Diner?"

I met Nikos and we ordered Eggs Benedict from Kyle, a once-gorgeous Australian who had also been stricken with AIDS.

Suddenly I noticed that Nikos's eyes had filled with tears. "Nikos, what's wrong?"

"I lied to you. I'm positive."

"Oh, God, I'm sorry Nikos. But you have to realize you can't blame me. It could have been anyone; let's face it, you've been with many people other than me. You can't blame anyone. I just want you to know that I love you with all my heart. You're the only one for me, always have been and always will be and when this thing is over, if it ever is, we'll be together again, I promise you."

Nikos walked me back to my apartment and as we said goodbye, we simultaneously handed each other copies of a Whitney Houston tape with the song "Didn't We Almost Have It All?" underlined. We'd both had the same idea—we both knew the lyrics were as if written just for us. Tears filled my eyes. How could something so perfect have ended like this?

"Nikos, I wish the best for you; take good care of yourself."

I rode the elevator up to my apartment feeling deeply lonely, as if half of me had been amputated.

It would be prohibitively expensive to have everything moved to California so I called *The Village Voice* to advertise everything from suits to furniture. I had one week to have everything moved out or be faced with the following month's rent.

Cindy and Spencer each took me out to dinner; other than that, there was no fanfare when I left. I took the Carey bus to La Guardia and looked back at the beautiful New York skyline reminiscing about everything that had happened there, wondering what kind of life, however short it might be, awaited me in California, and knowing that I would never have it all again.

Postscript

Having survived for over six years, James Melson lost his battle with AIDS on January 25, 1992 at a hospice in Los Angeles. He was 34 years old.

Epilogue

Back in 1959, when I was almost the same age as James Melson at the beginning of his autobiography, I remember going to see a technicolor melodrama called *A Summer Place*. I could barely drag myself home from the theater because it made me so depressed. It was at that point that I realized I was never going to be tall, blond, and handsome like Troy Donahue. For the rest of my life I was going to be a short, plain, Jewish man with eyeglasses, battling my tendency to be pudgy. (I didn't know then that I would also be completely bald by the time I reached thirty.) I don't think I was a troll; nobody ever threw me out of bed because of my looks. I was an ordinary-looking guy, but I suspect that Melson might have classified me along with Seymour Klein, who beat him out for a promotion, as a "quintessential Jewish geek" (p. 158). Having never fallen in love with my mirror as Melson did, it was a little hard to sympathize with the problems of a narcissistic "golden boy" as I read through his history. I've managed to face the same gay world without the benefit of the physical assets its denizens are expected to prize, but I've had my own wonderful time.

I, too, published an autobiography in my thirties (*Under the Rainbow: Growing Up Gay*, William Morrow and Co., 1977), but mine was quite a different story. The assets that I brought to gay life were different from Jim Melson's, but that never stopped me from getting my share of hot sex. For one thing, "golden boys" never turned me on. They never seemed quite real to me. I never believed that blonds had any more fun than the rest of us. They came out of that other America, where the corn grew tall and grim-faced men posed with pitchforks in front of the town church. They may have descended from German or Scandinavian or British immigrants, but they weren't usually called "Danish-American" or "English-American." They were simply "Americans," and as a Jew, I was the one with the hyphen, an exotic even in the exotic world of homosexuality. Like Melson, I was attracted to swarthy men with dark hair and eyes, preferably with mustaches or beards, and there were more than enough willing examples of those in my New York, where I moved as soon as I was able, so that I could be myself.

Also like Melson, I had been wounded by the unsympathetic world I had grown up in. Until recently, virtually all young gay people have had to make their way to self-acceptance alone. The bosom of the heterosexual family was the last place that most of us could look for understanding and support. But that journey from the disapproval and ignorance of parents, siblings, and childhood play-mates to the acceptance of homosexual peers is profoundly strength-ening for those who survive it — unimaginably so for those who never dare to embark on it. What Jim Melson never found was the affirma-tion and support that now abounds in the gay community. He lived in a thrilling time, but unlike so many people his age who participated in the gay liberation movement, he was not part of the gay history that was in the making. Melson was at a fringe of the action, which he mistook for the center because its yuppie values glittered so brightly. Beyond that fringe lay the isolation and loneliness of the closet, where much of the homosexual population lived apart from both the emerging gay political spectrum and the nightlife of the apolitical gay fast lane.

It wasn't until the months following the Stonewall uprising of 1969, at which gays fought back against a routine police raid and inaugurated the modern gay liberation movement, that I became a politicized homosexual. I joined the Gay Activists Alliance (GAA), whose meetings were soon drawing upwards of five hundred peo-ple. That was when I began to see the incredible range of personali-ties in the gay world.

Stereotypical gay men are expected to be flighty and irresponsi-ble, hypersensitive, and overemotional, inclined to aesthetic rather than mechanical matters, fashionable rather than political, un-athletic, promiscuous, permanently vain, and bitchy whenever pos-sible. The people I met in GAA may have been some of those things, but among them were construction workers and physicians, philosophy students and auto mechanics, athletes and loving par-ents, stoics and politicians, committed monogamists and occasional drag queens. Within the year I was elected secretary and then vice president of GAA, in both cases winning against men who were better looking than I was, and that taught me that in spite of what society thought, superficiality is not what all gay people are about. They liked me for my personality, my mind, my skills. (And a considerable number of them liked me for my sexual talents as well.) Narcissism may be one option for gay men, but it is not the only one. I chose another route.

Even during the years before gay liberation, when I had lurked in public men's rooms and skulked around the streets of Greenwich Village cruising for sex, hoping not to be recognized by someone from the college where I taught, I had never thought that what I was doing was wrong. Nothing that felt so good physically and so fulfilling spiritually could be evil. Nonetheless I had been ashamed because I had been taught that what I was doing was unmanly. I was hardly superficial or vain—certainly not as vain as the straight guys who combed their hair for half an hour at a time. It took communication with people like myself to assure me that what I was was okay.

Instead of the world of competition, one-upmanship and rejection that Jim Melson discovered, I found a world of mutual nurture and encouragement. Of course there were occasional sexual rebuffs, but I said no to men as often as they said no to me. All of our rejections, however, were gentle but firm, and happened early on. Once the foreplay had begun, it was considered poor form to throw someone out of bed simply because his dick was too small, as Melson did several times. Rarely have the confessions of a size-queen been more candid. His obsession with genital size even extends to the works of art in Florence's Uffizi museum, "perusing dickless statues and faking artistic awe. Obviously Michelangelo was unfamiliar with John Holmes" (p. 170). I visited Florence, too. My artistic awe was genuine, the statues' dick size notwithstanding, and I've seen films of John Holmes swinging his legendary endowment at jaded actors who were faking *sexual* awe.

The sensibility of the gay movement grew so politically hyperconscious that we were soon past the popular issues of sexism, racism, ageism and heterosexism. We were discussing the merits of "heightism," "ableism," and "looksism." Jim Melson, as obsessed as he was with appearance, would certainly have been indicted in the latter category, not to mention the ageism he reveals in the Cape Cod episode. At the bar there, he finds the clientele "long in the tooth," and when he is approached, albeit gracelessly, by "a portly, double-chinned, walrus-like Lothario," he pushes the man into the crowd, drenching everyone with their own drinks. "I can't take these old faggots. Get me out of here," he exclaims to his host, Spencer. He calls this "one of the most treasured moments of my life, for it was the first time I stood up for myself like a man." When he encounters the older gay couple, Harcourt and Lloyd, he is grateful that his relationships had ended early: "Who wanted to watch, embittered, as they succumbed to sagging paunches, arthritic joints, and wrinkled skin?" This is not a man who understands the meaning of love, and his affair with his mirror had not yet taught him to see himself. He berates his hosts for their overeating and alcoholism while he continues to overindulge in more fashionable drugs.

Of course, those whom he criticizes are hardly blameless themselves. Lloyd advises him to: "just keep it clean and stay away from those ethnics and exotics. God knows what kind of microbes they carry around" (p. 96). Melson even tosses in gratuitous anti-Semitic references for no apparent reason other than to illustrate the nature of his prejudices. In describing how awful the environment was at the meat packing plant where his father got him a job, he includes a portrait of Abe, a kosher slaughterer known as "The Rabbi," who is described as ". . . a giant of a man, about 6 1/2 feet tall and about half as wide, with a nose that could have vacuumed Nick's carpeting." Although he is utterly apolitical, his persistent references to the "Nordic perfection" he shares with other models have uncomfortable echoes of the blather about a "master race," which can still entice the politically naive into fascism.

The foundation of all these embarrassingly shoddy values is, of course, Melson's own self-hatred. He hated himself for once having been overweight, and he projects those feelings onto others: "My, I'd become particular! Being an ex-fatso made me no more tolerant, no less exacting and demanding. Quite the contrary: It was as though I'd turned onto others the critical scrutiny *I'd* received for years" (p. 41). But his early overeating is a common syndrome among gay men, a response to internalized homophobia. Near the end of the book, when he is befriended by Jane, he comments: "God, what I had missed in life by sacrificing what's really meaningful for the sake of the frivolous, the merely physical, the short-lived! If only I had not been possessed by this evil homosexual lust, Jane would have been prime life partner material" (p. 193).

Melson's narcissism and his prejudices, then, are little more than a thin mask for his feeling that being homosexual is an ugly, unnatural, immoral thing; and all his glittering experiences in the gay world—sex with beautiful men, dancing at chic discos, visiting glamorous places, being pursued by fashion photographers, mingling with famous and wealthy people—did little to enhance his feelings of self-worth. So he presents himself as everything that is wrong with gay male culture, wrapped up in one vainglorious package. Yet the man who wrote this life story is someone other than the main character in it.

It is only at the end of his story that we begin to see the impact of AIDS on the life he had thought was charmed. He regains his weight; he loses the man he loves; he discovers that illness has rendered him less attractive to others; his earlier terror at a temporary facial blemish which might ruin a fashion photograph is replaced by a permanent Kaposi's sarcoma lesion, a visible emblem of his mortality. Understandably unable to accept his new identity at first, he continues to project his self-hatred onto others when he asks himself at a support group for people with AIDS: "Did I now belong with this trash?" (p. 191).

Finally, his viewpoint begins to shift. Not surprisingly—I won't be cynical enough to say opportunely—he discovers religion. At long last, he performs an act of human kindness, giving sound advice and money for food to a young drug addict. It is not this single charitable act that redeems him. If anything, it is the writing of this autobiography that signals a sea change in Jim Melson. Presenting himself so frankly, warts and all, is an acknowledgement that he has come to see what was wrong with the way he treated other people and with the way he viewed himself.

What would this handsome young man have become had he not been stricken with AIDS? Allowing other men to wine and dine him, to house him and take him on expensive vacations solely because of his good looks, he had always been careful not to cross the line from exploitation of others to actual prostitution by refusing to provide sex for his benefactors. Would he have continued on his hedonistic path for another decade or two, trying desperately to fend off the ravages of age and retain his youthful looks, ultimately resorting to skin treatments and facelifts? Would he have enjoyed rejecting others sexually as long as he could, but eventually, furtively, been driven to pay hot young men for sex? Or would he have grown wiser and kinder with age and ultimately evolved into a "golden man" whose values were more than skin-deep?

There is no way to know what might have been, any more than there is a way to know what direction the gay world would have taken without AIDS. When gay politics and the sexual revolution coincided in the 1970s, a gigantic party was unleashed. Like Melson, I, too, enjoyed the playground that New York had become. I saw Bette Midler and Barry Manilow perform at the fabled Continental Baths, and I danced at The Saint and even once visited Studio 54. I spent summers on Fire Island, sometimes at the fashionable Pines, more often at the less sophisticated Cherry Grove, but it didn't matter because late at night the men of both towns met for egalitarian sex in the woods that filled the area between them.

For more than a decade, men who had grown up feeling isolated and inadequate were able to celebrate their special brands of sexuality with wild abandon. This carnival of the senses was born in the libido, not at a political meeting. Although it was possible to retain a basic sense of human decency at the orgy, politically correct sex—which had reached the point of saying that in the name of equality no one should be on top—was ignored in favor of the sort of sex that led to memorable orgasms.

Again like Melson, I, too, had a series of relationships—but the easier it was to get sex, the less trouble it seemed worth, and sex without emotional encumbrances was the order of the day. In the 1970s, gay men sought sex not with one particular person, but with "masculinity" in general, represented by the kind of male icons Melson danced with at Flamingo. Off the dance floor, these men were the "clones" who patrolled Christopher Street. Dressed uniformly in workboots and flannel shirts and leather bomber jackets, they semiotically advertised their sexual tastes with color-coded handkerchieves ostentatiously protruding from the back pockets of

their Levi 501s, in blatant disregard of the politically correct pro-
scription against sex objectification.

The further I went into this world, the less personal it became. It
was less threatening to trade the most intimate sexual fantasies with
men I didn't know at all. It began with frequently bringing home an
anonymous trick for sex and hoping he wouldn't stay for breakfast
and reveal that he was nothing like the fantasy man I'd had sex with
the night before. In time, I gravitated to the bathhouses like the St.
Marks and the Everard, and eventually to the back room bars like
The Mineshaft, where I could literally reach out and simply grasp
what I wanted. They were places at which Jim Melson would
doubtless have turned up his cute nose, but why would I have
cared? The men were hot, and I was having fun.

The fun had a dark side to it, however. Curiously, the sexual
settings grew to resemble the very scenes we had just liberated ourselves from. Some bathhouses erected complicated fantasy settings
so that customers could pretend they were in parked trailer trucks or
prison cells. Private clubs turned themselves into oversized men's
rooms. One place, The Glory Hole, specialized in cubicles with
holes cut in the wall, so that totally anonymous sex — not with a
man, but only with his genitals — could be facilitated. All our hard-
won freedom and community was leading us right back into the
arms of alienation and solitude. It's true that these places had a
warm sense of camaraderie, but there was also a coldness about
them, and as the political movement began to subside, the brotherhood in the bars and baths seemed comparatively superficial.

Even if our solidarity had been totally intimate, there was no way
to know that we were passing a deadly virus among ourselves. Once
the news began to emerge, it took several years before the implica-
tions of it began to sink in, and the sex palaces began to close,
either because of municipal force or from sheer loss of business.
Some of them were simply driven underground or reopened in new
forms a few years later. Safe-sex jerk-off clubs were formed, and
monogamy began to gain new respect, bringing with it a return to
emotional intimacy and the value of mutual nurture.

Sex, of course, could not simply disappear. It is a basic human
urge. Much of the younger generation has grown up with the rules
of safer sex already in place, so they regard condoms and the prohi-
bitions against certain sexual acts as normal limitations on their

behavior. The more daring among them, however, still flirt with disaster because they want to experience maximum sex. Like most young people, they secretly believe they are invulnerable and that bad things like illness and death will only happen to others. Some of them think they are safe if they have unprotected sex only with people under 25, forgetting that some of those people have had unprotected sex with older partners, and ignoring the statistics that say that the highest percentage of new cases is among people of their age group. Unsafe sexual practices have been reported in a number of new underground clubs, so the danger that the epidemic will continue to spread remains alive and well.

But for the generation of the 1970s, the carefree party was definitely over in the 1980s, and most of us were too busy nursing our dying friends to think about staying up all night on drugs for the sake of sex. With a serious look in our eyes, we joke that most of our socializing now is done at funerals and fund-raisers. I am one of the lucky ones. I have had a relationship for a decade now, and both my lover and I have tested negative for HIV. In the last ten years, I have seen more than 100 of my friends and acquaintances sicken and die, and more are yet to follow. But I have also seen a new generation rise up and take their places in volunteer service organizations like Gay Men's Health Crisis (GMHC) and political activist groups like the AIDS Coalition to Unleash Power (ACT-UP) and Queer Nation. They are angry and impatient, and they take for granted the freedoms won by my generation. Calling themselves "queer" rather than "gay," they are as impatient with the "gay" generation of the 1970s as we in GAA were with the "homophile" generation that preceded us.

All this has happened against a background of increasing erotophobia in America. Public passions have been stirred not only by the AIDS epidemic, but by epidemics, real or imagined, of child molestation and sexual harassment. Right-wing campaigns against pornography have been launched from the Attorney General's office. The National Endowment for the Arts has been pressured to defund gay-themed art. Fundamentalist religious groups have raised the battle cry against abortion, and with threats of economic boycott they have frightened the television networks away from depictions of homosexuality as anything other than a social problem. Concerned by the media's demonization of gay people during the AIDS crisis, I, along with several friends from the long-defunct Gay Activists Alliance, helped to found the Gay and Lesbian Alliance Against Defamation (GLAAD) in the mid-1980s. I'm proud to say that GLAAD has become an active force across the nation in fighting the ignorance that engenders negative portraits of gay people in literature, journalism, films, television, radio, and song lyrics. It is a battle that will be waged for some time to come, and in spite of the dark outlook of the present, I fully believe that it will eventually be won.

If a person like James Melson can grow from benightedness and self-hatred toward enough self-acceptance to present his life's journey as a role model of learning to be tolerant, America can grow out of its homophobic adolescence and learn an adult respect for the virtues of its own diversity. I don't need to treat the "golden boys" of our culture as a minority group oppressed by its own privileges in order to respect them as individual human beings as full of imperfection and aspiration as the rest of us. Each of us has a lesson to learn in life, and theirs has to do with overcoming their own beauty.

I remember a Sunday brunch seven or eight years ago when one of my friends brought along a handsome young man he'd been sleeping with. My friend was one of the first political leaders of the post-Stonewall gay movement, I was a writer and teacher, and with us was our friend Vito Russo, the internationally known lecturer on gays in film. I don't mean to be immodest, but the conversation at our table was genuinely interesting. The handsome young man never heard it, however. He spent the entire time transfixed with admiration of his own image in a mirror near our table. I was sorry for him, but I'm not sorry for Jim Melson. In writing this book, he shows us that he has learned a painful lesson well. It is not just a history of a glittering life. It is a history of human growth, for in writing it, he is offering a useful lesson to those gay people who will come after him, and that makes him—whether he knew it or not—a valuable member of our tribe.

—Arnie Kantrowitz
New York City, 1992